Nobody Lied

A Candid Chronicle:
Combatting Cancer

Roger A. Page

Dedicated To Difference Makers

Rodney Crowell wrote and sang:

Out on the road that lies before me now
There are some turns where I will spin
I only hope that you will hold me now
'Til I can gain control again.

That I have now lived those famous lyrics, and while at it felt the level hand of a strong and loving companion steadying us through each turn, never once failing to right the wheel when I couldn't, I find phrases like, "Thank you," or even, "I love you," to fall far short of the words I could search for forever and yet never find.

... But I'll say them anyway; Thank you, Karen, I love you.

Acknowledgements

I can see, now, how some of these Hollywood elites stand up there chewing at the air until the music drives them away. If I were to take their route in thanking or acknowledging everyone I should, my acknowledgements would equal the pages of this book. The handiest way to go about it is to assure you that the people to whom I owe the greatest thanks to for the outcome of this book show up on nearly every page. They in fact wind up being much of the *reason* for me to have written it.

For this particular book I did not seek a lot of help in editing, only my brother Ron along with my wife Karen read things over for me. Aside from a few minor tweaks each agreed things were in order, as they should be—after all there is only the barest truth to write about cancer. I hope, of course, to have given a fair depiction of the people involved, but as far as the cancer goes, this is not a book with elastic parameters like those I typically prefer to write. Those who know me understand I thrive on the poetic licensing granted authors in creative non-fiction—a classification of writing that demands an author must somewhat adhere to the truth... but really? I joke about it, but to me embellishment has never been out of the question when talking about my favored topics, hunting, fishing, landscaping, rural living, or redneck travels—particularly cruises. Sometimes during those wild rides I need to be reeled in a bit by volunteer editors caught in the act of rolling their eyes and shaking their heads.

But cancer is never going to subject itself to such fare. Cancer deserves to be told straight down the middle and I promise to have done that.

As far as acknowledgements go, I do thank my brother and my wife for their time spent and for their inspiring compliments. Besides those two, my sister-in-law, Cheryl, and a handful of others were quite integrally involved in my struggles, helpful whenever called upon. Beyond that, however, the best way to acknowledge the long list of deserving and wonderful people who have helped me make it this far is to go ahead and let them tell their own parts of the story.

Forward

At publishing, the jury is still out regarding my prognosis. But it will always be like that I guess unless or until it turns dire enough that my prognosis winds up terminal. I hope to never cross that bridge despite learning during this battle that I would be able to do it without undue complaint—of course if granted a choice I suppose I would opt to worry than to know. But it is clear to me that once a person starts with cancer they adapt a permanent shadow which will always lurk even in light of their ability to go on to live a happy extended life. This shadow, though, is only asking as much of a cancer patient as any human. All of us, cancer or not, must bury some demons along our way but we seem to function quite smoothly in spite of knowing those things about ourselves. Of course the telling difference is a person cannot simply suppress cancer; should it decide to reappear there is no burying it.

But until a patient's cancer is pronounced terminal, those of us who at first imagined the worst are often given chances to get back to tossing fishing lures, screaming at referees, camping in ground blinds, tending landscapes, hiking with our hounds, all of those things and more. As long as we can keep sidestepping the gravest perils of such a gripping disease, each of our breaths matter even more than they would have had we never been stricken. That's certainly not meant to applaud cancer, but to point out the chances for meaningful days beyond it.

Indeed, these days cancer does not translate to fatality nearly as often or at least as swiftly as it did not long ago, and that continues to improve. Had my life never come down to Doctor Sussman lowering the boom, I would never have been able to conceive the incredible technological tools or the unbelievable knowledge and skills that medical professionals are able to employ. It is, without exaggeration, a world full of brilliance in lockstep with elite expertise. If one must be a cancer patient we couldn't ask for a softer place to fall.

Having now seen it up close and placing my unmitigated trust in the hands of these pros I wonder what kind of world we might live in if all of us became so accomplished in our own chosen fields. I know as a professional landscaper who built a pretty solid reputation for knowing his stuff, I pale dismally in comparison to what these people put into play each day. I cannot begin to fathom the dedication and sacrifices these people made during their youth that formed the building blocks for them to become so exceptional. Millions of these professionals exist across the globe dedicating their lives so that little by little cancer slowly becomes more and more controllable and treatable.

This is my personal story about it. The people I have met, the support I have leaned upon, the inner truths—even those I had to fight against, many long days in self-induced seclusion, and now finally the recovery process where I currently advance... all of it so strange, surreal at times, but now adding up to perhaps a new chance at living with a graduated perspective. Obviously it is not a story I ever sought to tell, it is not a story I enjoyed telling at all; but I do feel better that it is told.

At sixty-three years old I was nicely settling into an early semi-retiree's life of tossing baits to perch, pitching articles to editors, lounging around on the deck with my devoted hound, hiking our local woods, tending my favorite landscape here at home, and still sustaining enough work so that I could enjoy blabbing with delightful customers from time to time; all the things a man could hope for had finally come true. This book comes along, then, to wallop the daylights out of the beginning of a happy ending. Who in a right mind would *want* to write it? But that's water under the bridge. Personal moaning won't change a thing and, anyhow, I'm not willing one bit to feel sorry for myself.

Cancer quite frankly, and it's no secret, is a sonuvabitch. But cancer, too, is a great teacher, at least of sorts. As I said, I am not about to applaud the disease, but after enduring the treatments necessary to fight back I will testify that I have met some of the finest people on earth. I have stared honesty and bravery eyeball to eyeball so intensely that those images are burned indelibly into my mind and heart; particularly knowing they are cast against a backdrop of inescapable fear. I have been introduced to the simple sounding phrase, "difference maker," a phrase when put into practice emphasizes a philosophy that is not simple at all—it can indeed change your life. I have been made aware of living and dying beyond any previous scope even though living and dying are matters I had previously thought long and hard about. There has rarely been need for discussion about it, but throughout my years I have developed a strong sense of spirituality through observance and reasoning. But at this entirely new level, staring face to face with the unknown, I saw a further challenge to verify that my prior conceptions ran deep enough. I wound up content in finding they do. I am satisfied beyond a doubt about my own appreciation toward living and my realistic acceptance about dying. I am more aligned and solidified in those principles now than ever before.

Currently, I await an upcoming CT scan to determine if lingering "activity" in a lymph node is simply residual scarring still visible under radioactive contrast or is it indeed cancerous activity that weathered the storm. The docs all agree it will likely prove inconsequential and this part of my battle should be put to rest. On the other hand, there is my own fragile mind that fears the worst.

I chose to end this book before knowing that outcome for one of two reasons.

One, I don't want to haul readers back a single solitary step toward the pit of hell which you will see enough of herein; or, two, if it goes the other way, I don't think it will ever prove wise to perform a victory dance when it comes to this stuff.

With cancer it is probably best to never declare victory or admit defeat. Neither seems advisable. I have been granted a wonderful life no matter when it ends, and I have also seen the darkest side of myself due to the wrath of this horrid disease. If, after having gone through what I have, my words can reach out to others to offer whatever form of compatibility we share, at the very least to let you know you are never alone in this, I will consider it a book worthwhile. But no matter how I try, I cannot hide the selfish truth that it is also a book I wish had never come about.

    I'm sure you understand.

Contents

Introduction

Hesitantly, I begin.

Shy of vulgar mish-mashes or grisly murders, some of what lies ahead are the most unpleasant words a person might read. Having no idea about any one individual's tolerance for discomfort I don't know what to tell you about reading this book; but I can assure you of one thing—you *should* read it.

As I indicated, in breaking from some of my past work, I am herein mandated to refrain from creative non-fiction, as cancer does not cater to creativity. Cancer is too strong to be messed with in that manner so I won't. I do promise to be blatantly honest and will try my best to inject humor and stay upbeat when merited; but don't expect an abundance of it. Still, when all is accounted for I truly believe you will be glad to have read this book.

It is generally a writer's endeavor to trumpet a luring introduction so fruitful that it pumps a reader full of encouragement and they simply cannot wait to get going. So if it seems foolish of me to be warning readers about what lies ahead, I hope I won't talk you out of coming along.

It seems reasonable for people who have survived their own scares, or some who are in remission, or maybe some who are currently engaged in full battle, to find interest in my story, but the ones I want to reach most of all are those who have lived their lives so far cancer free. I especially want to warn against the old adage, "Taking things for granted," because as clichéd as it sounds any one of you might end up like me. One day you are laughing it up with a buddy who wants you to come spend a week fishing later in summer, and the next day you are annoyed by a slight earache. The earache persists until it encompasses your whole neck and now your throat hurts, too, and that's when you discover the swollen lymph node. The fishing trip you were planning during the entirely normal life you were living is about to have the rug ripped from underneath it.

What the pages ahead will describe in detail is a harrowing journey through what nurse Karena and Doctor Collier each called the "pit of hell." The only good preliminary news came when Doctor Sussman said it isn't a death sentence—but "a life changer for sure," and in both cases what lie ahead for me turned out understated. Once treatments began, maybe even earlier, and for a long spell after they were over, time crept along at a snail's pace and what I can tell you about my own experience is I lost my voice entirely for two long months, stayed relegated to a sitting position in which to sleep for several months, could not taste or even swallow food for months on end—feeding myself through a tube inserted into my stomach, I was prompted to pump prescription drugs, even prescribed narcotics into my system, and instead of each day inviting the challenges of the workplace, or a new adventure on a weekend, the sole objective of each day became to make it through. Instead of everyday challenges, schedules, and agendas, a cancer patient undergoing treatments eventually whittles down to seeing nothing but days of survival that appear never-ending. Instead of future plans, a cancer patient no longer shuts the lights out at ten-thirty and crawls into bed for seven hours of comfy sleep, no, they sit alone in the dark and doze off for a few minutes here and there between the harsh coughing that they learn to stifle only by leaning way forward with elbows on knees and head bowed low. Jolted awake after ten or fifteen minutes there are often times when even the toughest and strongest of us succumb to tears. And the tears occur more often than we want to admit.

Maybe I can convince people who have never had cancer to begin living as if they *have* had it. So you see why even as I cast a caution flag out to you, I still urge you to come along.

In my own case I can wholeheartedly assure you that if I make it to the summit of the other side I will never during my remaining days take for granted a good night's sleep, a tasty meal, a long day fishing or hunting, and with whatever of my voice does return I will use it encouragingly more than critically. With any luck, I will turn a loathsome invasion into a blessing in disguise.

Sam is a Nuclear Medical Technologist skilled in PET CT imaging and before he had even guided me down the first corridor leading us toward his mobile scanning unit we learned we were both the same age and had each beaten alcohol addictions back in the day. His addiction had been so infringing he actually has the date he quit tattooed onto his wrist; mine was so infringing I have it tattooed in my brain—November Ninth, Nineteen-Eighty-Four.

If you are not familiar with a PET CT scan, it is essentially an ex-ray of most of one's entire body using an injected radioactive dye to highlight "areas of concern." I have heard it referred to as a "contrast" dye. Cancer cells show up green and today we would find out if I had any other occurrences besides the known cancer at the base of my tongue and in an adjacent lymph node. The patient lies on a "bed" of sorts and is passed into a large tubular scanner for some forty-five minutes. Prior to the scan the patient is reclined in an adjacent room for an hour to relax whereupon the body fully absorbs the dye. Sam already had a patient being scanned so as he prepped me we didn't have much time to chat. However, as he was injecting the dye into my veins he looked up and said out of the blue, "Ya know, I doubt this will make you feel any better, but I've been where you are."

I had no idea that was coming, and less of an idea as to how to respond, so I didn't.

Finally it came time for my scan and Sam and an assistant, Doug, positioned me on the bed and locked my arms down into a comfortable but stationary position and the scan began. Once it was over with I took time to ask Sam, "What kind of cancer, Sam?"

"Lymphoma," he said, "I'm in remission but I think about it every day."

He then stood up from his monitor, turned toward me, and more deliberately stated, "Cancer changes your life forever, buddy." Then he looked me in the eye, extended his hand, and said, "Good luck my friend." That quickly I could tell I was going to be in caring and honest hands. That part I got right.

The world of medicine is flabbergasting and particularly advancements made in technology are mind-boggling. My thirty-three radiation treatments were to be delivered based upon a 3-D configuration intended to consider every conceivable angle hoping to stay on target and do as little collateral damage as possible. Doctor Collier, an oncology genius, would begin fine-tuning my unique design exactly in accordance with the damage at the base of my tongue, the lymph node, and nearby areas where the cancer might potentially spread. If I'm remembering even closely, Doctor Collier told Karen and me that the profiles he could choose from to get in the ballpark were infinite; he would cull at least a hundred to start with.

"Usually that gets me where I need to be," he said.

From those one hundred ballpark profiles Doctor Collier was able to narrow it down to the closest to my situation and from there he could fine-tune the program to my exact needs. It is a laborious process that takes nearly eight hours on average and a process that utterly astounds me.

Head radiation nurse Karena, following some preliminary chatter during our initial meeting put it as I mentioned earlier: "We're gonna drag you through the pit of hell and back again, but we'll be with you every step of the way. You're going to beat this; I'm here to make sure of it."

Now let me ask you... having heard what I have said so far, are you beginning to see my reservations? But please, I beg of you to keep your eye on the ball enough to see that having gone through what I am going through, I should emerge fully confident to convince readers that any of us who put gusto into our lives and live life to its fullest are guaranteed a happy ending. Oh, sure, death awaits us all, but by the time you close this book, I want badly to believe you will do so with a higher perspective. Most of us are quite capable of determining our own happy ending; we just need to learn to look at it that way.

Although difficult chapters admittedly lie ahead, as I begin writing this the tide is beginning to turn in my favor during recovery so I am looking forward to some happier chapters, too. My final treatment was completed three months ago so things are looking up... finally. My hope is to end on a high note and thus far things look pretty positive. Currently I am scaling the mountain away from the pit of hell, gaining strength day by day, regaining hope to get back to at least a semblance of the life cancer tried stealing.

This book is my own version of cancer dictated by my own unique situation, diagnosis, and prognosis, so I won't pretend to suddenly be an expert. I will state my story and remind you that it comes from a man who once lived every day to its fullest and was off to a darned encouraging start to semi-retirement when the door was slammed in my face. I want you to keep in mind throughout this book and forevermore that tomorrow it could be *your* ear that aches just a bit, and as that ache persists it could be *you* staring eyeball to eyeball with a doctor telling you words you cannot believe you are hearing. That way, as long as it is *not* you, I can count on you to embrace each day, each swallow of food, each good night's sleep, each laugh, and each healthy breath, with all the vigor you can muster.

For the rest of your life, always, always, remember, anyone of us could be the next to discover what Sam says, "Cancer changes your life forever."

I originally wanted to open by contending that everyone who struggles with cancer has a unique and valuable story from which we can all benefit. But I have since come to learn that so many people have fought this battle, and so many have "survived" this peril, that mine will likely be one in a long line of, by now, trite chronicles. Face it, there is sadly nothing unique about cancer. Nonetheless, I decided to at least stow my own notes for my own purposes, a writer's disguise for the undeniable fact that we cannot help ourselves. No matter the topic, no matter how overladen with repetitive discussion, no matter the volumes upon volumes that precede us, we inherently proceed anyway as if ours might be the truest breakthrough. It is an odd quirk, I admit, but who am I to be the first on earth to resist it?

So, welcome to cancer. I hate knowing anyone ever has to hear those words, but millions of us do and by deciding to go ahead and write this book I ultimately hope it to be useful to anyone who reads it... and to me.

Ah, Semi-Retired At Last...

It seemed exactly as I had envisioned it; exactly as I thought it would be. On an invigorating April morning I lobbed another cast toward where a small stream empties into the lake and the depth rapidly drops to ten feet. My sinker made a gentle plunk, my drop-shot rig plummeted to the bottom where I immediately initiated an enticing hopping motion with my new rod and in no time at all felt the slightest tell-tale tick of another perch. So strange, these tiny ticks of the perch taking the bait—until you set the hook you have no idea if it's a slob thirteen incher or something far lesser... but it hardly matters when you have all day. Before it's over you will certainly have your share of jumbo perch to take home. At some point during the day you can sit eating lunch in your boat, gear stashed aside for a sec while you take a break and think that only a year ago this would be a day spent with a landscaping crew on a customer's property cleaning up debris left behind by winter.

What made this particular day specifically rewarding is I had landed into a bunch of larger perch and the boat was filling up quickly. Coupled with a glowing sun beaming high in the sky it dawned on me I was compiling a fine nucleus for a magazine article. The next perch ticked, I set the hook, and pulled it toward the boat. I reached for my iPhone so I could snap pictures and began playing the perch to flash its brightly striped sides atop the surface where the sun gleamed against the black and orange stripes. After capturing some can't miss shots I netted the beast and added it to the rest.

As is typical on this particular lake, the action dwindles by mid-day but by then I had turned my attention toward the sure-fire potential of my article. Shortly before noon I reeled up my line and began busily posing my seventeen jumbo perch in an array of backdrops that might make for captivating photo-support to help sell my article. I loaded all of them at once into my small net for a unique shot, I dumped them all into one massive pile between the boat seats and that seemed pretty cool, made better yet when I hoisted one of the larger ones up and featured it above the rest for a fun shot. Great stuff, but the instant I thought to line them up across the boat seat where they stretched from one side of the boat to the other I knew I had my money-maker. To strategically accent the setup I staged needle-nosed pliers, nail clippers, an aluminum handled net, two fishing rods, and even a couple opened bags containing the plastic baits to which the hungry fish had succumbed. The more helter-skelter I could arrange the setting to simulate a wild perch fishing day the better. The final scene captured it so convincingly that no editor in a right mind could resist. The shot was a classic, especially when you consider the old aluminum boat, my dad's hand-me-down gift from so many years ago as the main backdrop. After a dozen shots of the eye-grabbing setup I next chose the largest of the bunch, a pot-bellied toad nearing fourteen inches, and prepared for the ever popular selfie. I centered us in my iPhone monitor and positioned us to remove any glare or shadows and then took several shots of that pose, too. Convinced I had enough photo-support I returned fishing, but the action had stopped. I moved on to try a few more spots before reeling up and heading back to the launch.

On the way home I came up with my title and sub-title for the article: *Hop Shotting For Spring Perch—When It's Alright To Fish The Drop-Shot All Wrong.*

Perfect.

To quickly explain, there is a popular bass fishing rig called the drop-shot. Nifty rig, too. There is a sinker on the bottom, and a foot or two above it, using what is called a Palomar knot you tie a hook that remains horizontal. Attach any small plastic bait onto the hook and it sits weightless hovering a short distance off bottom. Bass can't resist it so I thought why not perch. At first I struggled with the rig. From what I had read, the way to catch bass with it is to remain nearly stationary and to subtly wiggle your rod tip barely moving the bait. When I tried that with perch I failed to roust a bite. After a couple hours I grew frustrated and for the heck of it began to lightly jerk the rig along bottom. I have no idea what compelled me to do that, so here we have a prime example of dumb luck because I hadn't moved the bait ten feet before I felt the slightest little tick at my rod tip. Shocked, I rallied in time to set the hook on an eleven inch perch. Muttering excitedly, I chucked my rig back out into the water, repeated the hopping motion, and another nice plump keeper caved. The action persisted until I wound up with thirteen brutes on the very first outing. Since then the technique has worked time and again prompting me to jokingly rename it the hop-shot rig—why not?

Back to the day I was telling you about, I could not have been more confident in my article. I was right, too. The editor of the first magazine contacted, Fur-Fish-Game, said, "You bet, let's run it." When the article appeared it was supported nicely by the classic photo of the perch lined across the boat seat as well as a proud selfie and an informational side-bar I had constructed to reveal the baits and how to rig them.

Who could blame me in my euphoria to believe semi-retirement would be nothing but pure joy?

I spent my livelihood operating my own landscaping business and from mid-March until early December each year the schedule ranged anywhere from rigorous to torrid. I am not here to talk much about those days, but I can tell you this—standing on the finished end of thirty-one years is a sobering testament to the old adage about how time flies. I had not planned on taking my early retirement, hadn't given it much thought at all, until one evening during the off season before my sixty-second birthday, Karen, presented me with some figures she had dug up on my behalf.

"You might want to go to the Social Security website and check things out," she suggested.

I did that and soon after seeing the numbers in front of me I intensely tapped away at my calculator and when I ran the final numbers to find out it would take me seventeen full years to make up the difference in payments between early and normal retirement I could feel a dumb grin etching across my face.

The next thing to do was to draw up a form letter to customers to thank them and to give notice of my decision to step down from the landscaping duties. In that letter I made it clear I planned to continue performing lawn care in the form of fertilizers, organics, lime, and weed control. Years ago I had incorporated that service into my program having no pre-conceived plan but as it turns out, what an ideal supplemental income to a semi-retirement situation. In New York State, as I presume most other states, the government found their way into everyone's pocketbooks by demanding that businesses applying pesticides, even OTC herbicides, must become certified. That, of course, narrowed customer's choices on who they could hire to perform that work. Most landscapers haven't a clue about those sorts of things but I had plenty of experience and decided to use the government's greed to my own advantage and became registered. Since then the government has stayed a perpetual pain in the neck and charged me thousands of dollars in "fees" and "licenses," but in spite of that the lawn applications have paid tremendously over the years. As a supplemental income to my monthly SS payments I could make a go of things.

I think some of the happiest days of my life occurred the following springtime when in March and early April instead of heading off to work I towed my boat here and there and broke out the hop-shot on cooperative perch; then in mid-April I rekindled a nostalgic fondness for bullhead fishing—especially at night.

Once summer came along I set my fishing gear aside for a while and spent most mornings out on our deck with hound Audrey where we lazed about in the sunrise until I had finished my second cup of coffee. I no longer had mornings ruined by what I might have to say to such and such an employee today, or having to take a truck into the shop and work the day shorthanded, or listening to workers moan about the heat, and there are a million etcetera's I could come up with if need be.

But need not be.

No, sitting out there with Audrey anyone could tell that each of us were as carefree as the other. Around ten o'clock I might tend to some pruning or trimming on my own landscape, maybe work up the beds a bit, and after lunch I could mow the lawn whether it needed it or not. Such is the structure of semi-retirement—something I had labored toward for my entire life.

As far as work goes, there were periods where lawn applications needed to be timed.

Mid-April to Mid-May, late June through Independence Day, late August through Mid-September, and a couple of shorter blasts in October and November. Rarely would any working day comprise more than five hours.

What a wonderful place in life to be. At sixty-two years old and in robust shape, you can imagine how much I looked forward to my upcoming years...

Lowering The Boom

It began as an innocent earache in mid-May and the pain increased enough over the days that I began using a heating pad at times. Not a big fan of rushing to see what doctors think, I toughed it out in hopes it would eventually dissipate and go away. Instead the pain increased to encompass my neck and throat until one evening I ran my fingers across my neck to feel the obvious protrusion of a lump—a swollen lymph node for sure.

"Uh, oh, Karen," I blurted loud enough so she rapidly appeared from the kitchen to see what was wrong. "I think I'm in some trouble, here. I have a lump in my neck that must have something to do with the earache. I need to schedule an appointment with Sarah."

"Are you sure?" asked Karen, not wanting to believe a word I had said.

"Yeah, this isn't going to be good," I said, and I truly did know at that very moment that my future was in immediate jeopardy.

Karen works as a medical records clerk in the same office where my personal choice for a physician, a nurse practitioner named, Sarah, is located. Karen made the appointment for me the following day.

Sarah felt the lump, agreed it was a severely swollen lymph node and scheduled an ultrasound. The ultrasound led to a CT scan and the CT scan led to Sarah calling me at home to say she was referring me to an ENT specialist, Doctor Sussman,

"He's very good," promised Sarah, "You'll be in good hands."

The trip to Doctor Sussman's office found my mind awhirl. I already knew what was coming but knew zilch, of course, about any specifics. It would be cancer, that much I was sure of, but beyond that would the magnitude of it mean that within this very hour I would hear news telling me to prepare to die? Maybe it would be as simple as scheduling a quick in-and-out day surgery where they merely remove the lymph node and send me on my way. One thing for sure, it was not a pleasant ride.

At Doctor Sussman's office the nurse escorted me into a room where Doctor Sussman sat at his computer working on another case.

"Have a seat, I'll be right with you," he said, hardly looking up at me, and I sensed a shortness in his voice that indicated perhaps a callousness that doctors, doing this day in and day out, might unconsciously submit to. Patients, on the other hand, sit there on pins and needles waiting for confirmation that our lives are about to forever change. I found his mannerisms a bit cold, but I wasn't here to make friends so sat quietly on my pins and needles.

When he at last did swing his chair away from his monitor he motioned me toward a large reclining chair and said, "Sit here."

Next he retrieved what I have since learned is called an endoscope—a microscopic camera slid up one of your nostrils to gain information about what is going on in the throat. To some, I guess this nasal endoscopy is tolerable, but I am not one of those.

"I need to take a look," said Doctor Sussman. "This might be a little uncomfortable but it won't hurt," and that quickly he was shoving his endoscope up my nostril. I had nothing to do with my reaction, no control whatsoever as I drew back involuntarily at the horrible invasion.

"I need you to relax," he said, and that sounded like, "lots better than being shot in the nuts, ain't it?" I must have hung tough enough for him to get what he needed and when he at last slid the endoscope back out of my nostril he handed me a Kleenex I guess I had earned.

I have since learned how essential the endoscope is to an ENT specialist, and I truly want to make their work as easy as I can, but I can assure you, too, that some reactions are out of our immediate control. I hate endoscopes with a passion and doubt one will ever get past me again despite my wanting to cooperate.

He undoubtedly gained enough information, though, because after a quick evaluation over at his computer he slid his chair back over to me, looked me directly in the eye, and said, "I'm afraid I have to lower the boom a bit, here" and I heard myself gasp desperately.

The first words you hear are, "You are going to die," which is how I interpreted "lower the boom." Doctor Sussman described carcinoma on the left base of the tongue and in the adjacent lymph node. He then scheduled a biopsy to confirm his diagnosis, but told me he was absolute about what he had seen.

I asked if he thought the cancer would be treatable and he said, "Oh, yes, by all means. I'm not giving you a death sentence here, but it's a life changer for sure."

I would come to find out he wasn't kidding.

The ride home was a numbing half-hour of wondering what now. I opened the door at home, patted Audrey on her soft head and

36

when she gazed up affectionately I stifled some tears while sitting down next to her.

"Dad's gonna have some rocky times ahead, sweetie," I said.

When Karen came home I didn't try to ease into anything, it isn't how we do things, I simply said, "It's cancer."

"You're kidding," she replied.

"Not kidding, Kare. It's on the left base of my tongue and in the lymph node."

She turned silent, headed into the kitchen to put some groceries away, changed from her work clothes, gave Audrey an affectionate pat on the head, we ate dinner, watched TV, and then she cried half the night away after I had somehow fallen asleep.

Coming Out With It

My biopsy was scheduled a few weeks out. What had begun in May had now stretched into July. I had remained silent but now that the diagnosis was clear I leaked it to my neighbor who optimistically replied that the biopsy will probably prove benign.

"No," I told him, "It's not benign"

I then asked that he keep it under his hat so I could let people know on my own terms as things unfolded.

When Karen learned I had talked it up with the neighbor she was not happy.

"Wait until you know for sure what the deal is," she said.

"I already do," I insisted, but I knew she was right.

I will tell you this, though, cancer is as hard to stay silent about as it is to come out with.

When the biopsy confirmed Doctor Sussman's original diagnosis, what I had known since mid-May, I decided it time to let others know what I was up against.

There is always plenty bad to say about social media, but plenty good to say about it, too. In this case, I could let over two hundred people know at once about my plight; that as opposed to it leaking out in whispers of, "did you hear about Roger Page..." I took a great deal of time to word my Facebook post exactly as I wanted it put. Too often I have watched responses to news like this sloughed off with a tearful emoji, or a hurried, "sending prayers," or worst of all, that emoji of the praying hands. The English language supplies us with a dictionary several inches thick full of words for us to select from at times like these. It was important to me, at least in this case, that my affliction toward words, as well as my personal assessment of faith, be respected.

After writing, editing, re-reading, editing, and re-reading, I shrugged my shoulders and said, "here goes," and posted it. Here is how it read:

I guess it's time to talk out loud about some challenges I am readying to face. All I ask is after hearing me out you treat me no differently than you did yesterday. We all contend hurdles; I've jumped my share, so count on me to dust this one too.

In May I discovered a swollen lymph node in my neck and told Karen, "I think I'm in some

39

trouble." I was right. After several hospital visits, ultra-sound, cat-scan, and biopsy, the current diagnosis is, "carcinoma of the left tongue base and adjacent lymph node." Tomorrow I will learn more definitively about the road ahead, but the doctor hinted to Kare that the next step will likely be a PET CT scan to determine if there are other areas to address, and if that goes well it looks like some intense radiation treatments and probably some chemotherapy sessions loom to try to eradicate the localized cancer.

I want to talk personally with you for a minute, but before I do, allow me to ask a favor. Please do not respond to what I am telling you with tearful emoji's, praying hands, and the like. The English Language is so richly abundant with meaningful words of encouragement and they speak far more optimistically than fear, sadness, or desperation, none of which are in order here. Even if you say nothing at all I will consider you to be in my corner, but if you do have words of encouragement, by all means now would be a great time to spit 'em out.

Political news mogul Charles Krauthammer lamented in his last days that he was sad to leave this world but had "lived the life I intended." At the same time Charles was saying goodbye is when my cancer was confirmed by an ENT specialist, Dr. Sussman, who looked me squarely in the eye and said, quote: "I guess I have to lower the boom a bit here."

Even though I suspected cancer from the get-go, it still takes your breath away to hear it verified. But once it sunk in and the doc comforted me by adding, "Look, it's not a death sentence, but it is definitely life changing," I turned again to Krauthammer's pragmatic advice. Having survived an accident rendering him to a wheelchair, Krauthammer went on to help others by telling us that only by our full acceptance of what befalls us will we overcome it. He was correct and I live on as proof.

At the same age Krauthammer was accepted into Harvard I was a reckless kid exhibiting such destructive behavior I wound up in jails at times, underwent psychiatric evaluation, and eventually needed to convince a probation officer I could straighten things out. I can see jaws of people who know me these days dropping to learn of it; it is not something I have ever talked about. Then, in 1984, my oldest brother, a man I idolized, was killed in a one-car accident near San Francisco. Jake never acknowledged his alcohol addiction but the horrible event signaled me to expect the same fate. I already had a couple of close calls and in November of that year when a cop pulled me over I decided to fully accept alcohol as a demon and to rid it from my life.

Thanks to that victory I was at last able to put Krauthammer's phrase—living the life I

41

intended—into motion. And since then, if anyone has ever lived a wonderful life it is me. I am never sure I deserved all the good things that have come my way, but I have always done my best to seize each day positively and even in light of these recent findings vow to continue.

As far as this cancer goes I could not be in better hands and for my own part, every single nurse, doctor, and person who already knows of this has outwardly championed my attitude as they should—after all, with their help I have no reason to carry doubts.

Finally, Kare has worked for Guthrie Medical now for nearly thirty years. She never moans about low wages (except to be insulted by McDonald's workers needing $15 per hour— that did piss her off, I admit), she has "blasted" out of our driveway through fallen snow in wintertime, she has worked Sundays on occasion to "get some overtime," and she wouldn't dream of taking days off frugally. She is a continuous beacon of light and despite what she is paid hourly, so far I have been obligated to pay about sixty dollars or so while receiving thousands upon thousands of dollars' worth of care because my wife carries medical benefits that cover me head to toe. Because of all she does, and how much I love her, I elect her to be Captain of my team moving forward... but I do prefer that docs and nurses take care of the heavier lifting if you don't mind.

Okay, that's off my chest.

Thanks for being my friends. Share if you think anyone on your own friends list needs to know any of this, and most of all, whether this is just a blip in the road or ultimately a showstopper, nothing will alter the final result that I feel exceedingly lucky to have emerged into the life I intended.

After posting it I obviously worried about offending some people about the faith thing, but in this case I did not want to encourage them, either. Religion has nothing to do with cancer, yet while I have continually seen prayers levied every single time cancer is mentioned I have kept my mouth shut... but not this time.

Luckily I have earned respect from most of my religious friends who know me to be as compassionate and giving as any human can be. I never judge them or argue with them about their beliefs and won't ever. Most of them are kind hearted souls that truly trust in faith; I am a kind hearted soul that bears no allegiance whatsoever to faith. In this case I was relieved that few chose to make an issue about my request and fewer yet went ahead and overrode it. I knew there would be some, of course, but for the most part friends took time to find actual words of encouragement and heartfelt thoughts. It was uplifting and humbling to read their compassionate and inspiring comments.

With the news now out and having been met with a resounding response of support echoing back, along with my full acceptance of what had befallen me in order, I gave in and openly cried. I would come to learn over the next months that cancer brings along with it a lot of tears... and fear.

Faith, Prayers, And The Killdeer

I cannot think of a single person who knows me that would tell you there is a chance in hell I'll wind up in hell. If that person exists, they have kept their feelings well hidden. But here is how that works. Back to Charles Krauthammer, when he ascertained that while some people are borne to faith and some are not, the farthest off base are atheists, he described the feelings of a lot of us. Yes, we refuse to subscribe to a God a Heaven and a Hell to universally explain our life's purpose, but we are every bit as spiritually inclined as any devoted person. Krauthammer never once shied from his posture on faith—he simply could not subscribe to it. His Jewish parents had given him plenty of background to work with but never forced the thought process in any certain direction. Charles figured out at a young age that he was not a man of faith. But nobody in a right mind would consider Charles Krauthammer a heathen. He was a deeply reflective person and passionate about a world around him governed by an explicit power. He did not need to be able to explain it in order to recognize it.

The minute Krauthammer passed, fellow newscaster Brit Hume offered a solemn eulogy in which he casually brushed off Krauthammer's views about faith. In fact Hume simply went ahead and assured everyone that God would certainly not want to be without Charles up there by his side. Hume, assuming the authority to grant Charles a pass, can now rest blissfully contented to know Charles is in Heaven despite Charles saying right out loud throughout his entire lifetime that he did not advocate God, Heaven or Hell.

So you see how it works.

That is exactly how prayer works. Please do not get defensive until you hear me out and I mean entirely out. This is not an easy subject.

As far as prayers go, they are boundless in making those who endorse them feel better about things. A person gets cancer, their friends bless the person with prayers. The person gets better—prayers work. The person does not get better—but they are in a better place, their suffering is now over, prayers work. Surely you can see why some of us raise our brows.

Bear in mind I am not a heathen. As a person who has sincerely contemplated religion and prayer every bit as much as anyone else I do believe higher powers govern our purpose. But I would be surprised if the complexities to our existence even approach the outer edges of human understanding. While humans continue to compile enviable knowledge about how the universe and beyond works, why would we not consider that perhaps the complexities of our own being are not yet within our grasp to figure out? Furthermore, why would we need to?

In my own case, I intentionally worded my Facebook post to prompt respondents to actually talk to me. That would help me a great deal at that point as I, along with Karen, had shouldered most of the entire burden ourselves for nearly two months. In an admittedly selfish sense, seeing prayers as extraneous gestures, I wanted to hear words that mattered. The truth is I understand prayer does no harm and in fact is a form of nicety to be appreciated. I get that. But what I needed to hear were tangible words; words I could actually *feel*.

As far as my cancer goes I am absolute the outcome will be contingent entirely on the skills of doctors and nurses versus the inevitability that sooner or later we die. If my particular prognosis holds true, the HPV virus

47

is treatable, my original PET CT scan proved clean besides the known cancer at the base of my tongue and lymph node, so chances are good for me to emerge in decent health. If that does come to pass I expect to hear my share of "prayers work!" I'm not complaining; it's a day I look forward to. But in reality it was *people* who invented the PET CT scan, Ultrasound, the 3-D Radiation Bed, and it was *people* who went to medical school for years and years and have since developed a vaccine for the HPV virus. Whenever cancer is beaten back and a patient is granted more years, it is because *people* work. The reason life-expectancy continues to expand is because *people* work.

I am sure I have printed it in other books, but this being the most outspoken I have been on the subject I want to say again that this life we are living should be miracle enough. The book I commonly refer to is called, *Unweaving The Rainbow*, by Richard Dawkins. In it he points out, "*We are going to die, and that makes us the lucky ones.*" Dawkins, wanting to substantiate Mervyn Peake's insistence that, "*To live at all is miracle enough,*" compellingly solidified his point; "*The potential people who could have been here in my place but who will in fact never see the light of day outnumber the sand grains of Arabia.*"

I sat with Karen out on our deck a few days after Doctor Sussman lowered the boom and we admired what we have done with our property, we reflected on cruises we have taken, we laughed at our raucous Seattle vacations cheering the Seahawks in the loudest stadium on earth, we laughed all the way back to a time in our lives when we were so poor we stood in a grocery store unable to afford everything in our basket. Reluctantly we agreed we would have to do without the cheese and we put it back. As I put it back I looked at Karen and embellished a solemn vow, "Someday we will be able to afford cheese," I announced right out loud. "I guarantee it!" and I emphasized my boast with a hearty fist pump. We left the store giggling over my clowning, but just a few years later it became a Christmas tradition for me to buy for her the most expensive cut of Norwegian cheese our nearby Wegman's grocery store would stock. As we sat together on the deck rehashing good times each of us took turns scratching Audrey's ears and when it turned silent I closed my eyes and continued inwardly with more personal memories. I reflected on hundreds upon hundreds of hours in the local woods, smelling the pines and woodstoves, listening to the scattering leaves falling down, trusting a misty rain or new snow to bring a deer within range, but if not, there was still the tranquil woods. I have spent as many hours, I guess, on nearby lakes and even the rumbling Ontario streams up north chasing this or that species of fish—and especially I have always lay in wait for a howling wind on a cloudy winter day to cast lures off Keuka Lake's shoreline and fight the gallant trout that live there. From the woods and the lakes arose over twenty nationally published magazine articles and that number continues to grow. I even drifted back to good times when a long-haired kid with a corduroy cowboy hat tore up the beer joints around here with a five-piece band. Lastly I relived some of the fondest moments of thirty-one years running a lucrative landscaping business and when I opened my eyes back up I turned toward Kare and caught her studying me. We have been in love a long, long time and seeing the worry in her eyes I reached to touch her soft hair and told her, "No matter what happens, I've lived a terrific life."

I am not a grain of sand, I am a breathing person enjoying his miracle for however much longer it lasts. Throughout my adult life while molding and cultivating my beliefs, it occurred to me a long time ago to leave religion out of it.

Increasingly, humans are evolving to question our mortal obsession with "everlasting" life. As a result, religious faith no longer stands by itself simply because of itself. It is no longer enough to assume a God waits to judge us, particularly a powerful yet loving God. I almost hate myself for saying it this way, but considering the untiring destruction being caused daily and worldwide in the *name* of religion it seems plausible to ask why a powerful yet loving God wouldn't possess enough relevance to work in less mysterious ways.

Is there any chance at all that humans simply haven't evolved to a point where we can understand what dictates our being? For a clear thinking human to come to a conclusion that a God, Heaven, and Hell, are probably not adequate to support the possible intricacies that encompass our universe surely seems reasonable. At least give those of us who question faith the benefit of the doubt that we are not doing it without having given things a lot of sincere thought.

The Killdeer

Not long ago I visited an immense garden nursery to grab some shrubs for some work around my own property. An employee, Ethan, escorted me about the vast premises in a golf cart in order to round up the shrubs I needed. At one stop he asked, "Hey, have you ever seen a killdeer?"

"A what?"

"A killdeer. It's a bird."

"I guess I haven't," I said.

"Follow me, you gotta see this," he said and led us a few steps down the stoned pathway where our encroachment induced a bird to suddenly burst from nowhere and zoom out ahead of us where it hadn't made it twenty full yards before it began flopping and fluttering about while screeching in sudden agony. It looked and sounded horrible. From its desperate wailing one surmised a bird in a terribly dire state.

"Holy smokes," I gasped, "It's in bad shape."

"No, not at all," said Ethan. "We're standing close to her nest and she's trying to draw us away. It's how they lure predators away from the nest. Isn't it cool?"

I headed toward her, faking further chase whereupon the mother killdeer suddenly rallied and scampered ahead, but the instant I again stopped she resumed feigning her tragic plight.

"That is something," I said, returning back to Ethan and our golf cart.

"We're within ten feet of her eggs," said Ethan, once I got back to him. "See if you can spot 'em."

Seeing no place nearby that should harbor a bird's nest I shrugged causing Ethan to grin and walk me over to four eggs lying prone, on the ground of all places, but looking so convincingly similar to the number two stone where they laid fully exposed you would never notice them without having reason to look. The eggs were so perfectly camouflaged the site needed to be marked with a small wired flag so the rest of the staff would know to steer clear. Even more astounding, though, was to learn that once the chicks hatch they are already adorned with a protective downy covering and can walk off the nest and find shelter the instant the feathers dry. If that was not the case, all the trickery in mom's playbook would fail in the long run.

When I echoed Krauthammer's perception that we needn't be able to explain something in order to recognize it, who cannot see what the killdeer is telling us? Lacking any logical empirical process, the killdeer's inherent behavior coupled with such fortunate conditions at birth surely seems outside the realm of natural selection. A female killdeer knowing to distract predators by feigning injury is not a result of luck, reasoning or anything in between. Doubled by the condition of her newborns allowing them to engage in their own preservation it is not naïve for one to claim a higher power is helping the killdeer along. If it's God, the logical question becomes why not grant the poor killdeer a nice protective tree like all the other birds get? By observing behavior that cannot possibly be learned, yet must be employed, and then seeing it universally applied among an entire species, makes any assessment insisting nothing but science or evolution is in play seem inept.

I chose killdeers due to the recentness of events, but really could have gone with any number of others. On our own property robins annually build nests and for years I gave it little thought. But one year a robin built her nest in a Hinoki Cypress directly below our bedroom window from where my wife and I enjoyed a bird's eye view of the whole show. It went on for weeks and as the process unfolded I understood how inadequate science and evolution are in trying to explain some of what occurs right in front of our eyes. To begin with, how does a robin know to begin a nest in the first place, how does it set about building it, and why are the results of every robin's nest essentially identical to all the other robin's nests even though no one robin has ever observed another's nest? But if you tell me God did this, tell me why, after all the time the mother has spent building the nest, nurturing her eggs and protecting her hatch, do please tell me why my cat, more than once, has climbed up to kill the birds for reasons unknown.

So, yes, I think there is a lot wrong on both sides when it comes to religion versus evolution and science. Until someone can convince me otherwise, the behavior of killdeers and robins satisfy me that to live this one life as the miracle it is and to ask nothing beyond makes the most sense.

To Those Who Pray

What I know best about those who pray is they are trying to convey positive thoughts and it takes an insensitive nitwit to condemn that aspect of it. Because I possess no animosity over people's religious beliefs or their trust in faith I should never use prayer as criteria when it comes to friendship. And I don't; I never have. I keep and enjoy the company of any number of friends devoted to their faith and I never feel compelled to change their thinking. But I do insist they respect my thinking. Those who know me understand that although I won't pray and cannot accept conventional faith, it in no way suggests I lack spiritual convictions at least equal to their own.

A post in the form of a religious meme made its rounds recently on social media.

When I say I'll pray for you, it isn't because I'm forcing my religion on you. It's because I believe in God and the power of prayer, and just because I care.

I see nothing at all wrong with that spirit of prayer, but if you really care, learn the *words* to say it. Joining the rank and file who so casually fire off the quick, "Praying for you," does not sound nearly as caring as when somebody takes time to use the incredibly abundant English Language to form a personal and meaningful sentiment.

Grateful Either Way

However it turns out for me, I am grateful for the life I have been granted and satisfied I have lived the life I intended. Should I beat this current cancer, sooner or later there will come a foe I will not beat. The same, of course, holds true for you. Death is inevitable so fearing it is irrational. But for now, as I go about my battle, at any juncture where victory is at least temporarily claimed, or else doom is foreseen, I will be trusting in medical experts and technology. Throughout this awful trek I have already been guided by some of the most astute people I have ever met. I can tell you with certainty given the incredible knowledge these doctors and nurses have accumulated in their profession, coupled with the mind-boggling advancements in medical technology, my fate is in capable hands and that's good enough for me.

Contending Barriers

Being A "Difference Maker."

Jim Kelly, the Hall of Fame NFL quarterback, besieged by an oral cancer that robbed him of some of his speech stays undeterred in routinely making his rounds on the speaking circuit anyway. There is much more to his story, though. Besides his own dreadful bout with cancer, his young son, Hunter, was diagnosed with globoid-cell leukodystrophy (Krabbe disease) and died of it when he was just eight years old. Kelly and his wife, Jill, have since propelled *Hunter's Hope Foundation* to help others in that same horrible situation, and there are many.

If you ever want to see a heartwarming moment it was when Kelly addressed some of today's NFL stars among a throng of other sports celebrities at the 2018 ESPY Awards. Kelly received the Jimmy V Award which commemorates valiant efforts carried on by ambassadors of cancer, and Kelly has certainly turned out deserving of such accolades. His emotional speech urged all within earshot to "Make a difference today for someone who is fighting for their tomorrow."

In an emotional appeal, Kelly emphatically pleaded to the illustrious audience before him. Broken tongue be damned, his words sent every last cheek streaming with tears.

"You don't *have* to be an Aaron Rodgers or a Russell Wilson to inspire someone and be a difference maker!" demanded Kelly forcefully, beseeching everyday humans to be "difference makers" at any possible juncture. Whenever you can be the one with the uplifting smile or kind gesture do not fail that opportunity. Be a difference maker every day all the time.

I have watched the video several times, and am determined to carry Kelly's advice forth. I have found that being a difference maker not only helps you inspire others, but it ends up being self-inspirational as well; win—win. Every single time you seize a chance to be a difference maker is another step toward realizing you are becoming a better person. It is gratifying as all get out.

And it works.

Sandra, an accomplished oncology nurse practitioner, oversaw and monitored my recovery. She was quite personable in more than a generic way, but she had patients besides me on her busy schedule so I wouldn't expect to chat it up like old friends at a reunion. But during one of my visits, Sandra sat quietly reviewing my bloodwork when I asked, "Hey Sandy, have you ever gone through any of this yourself?" Immediately she casually dropped her guard, put down her pen for a moment, and looked me squarely in the eye. "Not me, personally," she said softly, "but yes. People in my family and others very dear to me have fought cancer at one point or another." As her pen remained idle atop the desk between us she took a couple of minutes to talk outside the lines about cancer. Then before getting back to work on my charts she wanted to know more about this landscaping book I was finishing work on. She revealed her own penchant for gardening and, albeit for only a short time, Sandy seemed happy to drift over to her everyday human side for at least a minute or two that afternoon. I hope so.

I tried to do that with all the doctors and nurses when I could. There is often a built up guarded barrier between people in given situations. I felt it often as an employer versus my employees and it felt the same now as a patient versus medical pros. On both sides of the barrier are everyday humans and I have always subscribed to the notion we work better together as everyday humans than we do when saddled by our supposed roles. Outwardly, I believe it is probably part of a natural process that many medical experts seem to treat patients as the next in line, but how could you blame them? They are not here to solve how your kid did at little league practice or to hear the funny story about your camping trip last weekend; they see a human with something wrong with it that needs to be fixed. But bear in mind the possibility that doctors and nurses might have kids in little league, too, and perhaps they have funny camping stories, too. I learned right away the natural barrier between us needn't lurk as formidable as imagined.

Nurse Karena carries a no-nonsense reputation around the Corning Cancer Center and she likes it that way. But Karena can belly-laugh with the best of them if you get her human side going. Right off the bat she wanted to prepare me for what lay ahead during my upcoming treatments. As she prepared me she seemed redundant in warning me how tough she was liable to be. Well, hell, I'm an old football coach, "old-school Rog" was my nickname throughout the local landscaping circuit, so what do I care? I interrupted her, finally, and said, "Look, Karena, here's the deal. You have full permission to say to me whatever you want to say, and you can kick my ass with both boots if need be... which is exactly what I'm about to do to *you* if you keep calling me Mr. Page." From that point we were no longer a nurse and a patient, but two everyday humans working toward a common goal. Karena does take a tough stand at her job, that's why she is so accomplished at it, but she also has the wisdom to see in others that same toughness and I found her to be more of a cheerleader in my progress than I ever thought her to be a taskmaster. But toward the end of my treatments, at a point I admittedly hung by a thread, Karena was the one keeping her eagle eye on me while never once getting in my face about my dwindling attitude and my sullen demeanor. She knew, like I knew, I could make it across the finish line; but in case we were both wrong about that, Karena stayed ready to catch and drag my ass across if need be. She handled me like the consummate professional she is, and I trust I can speak for her in saying we knew, going in, we would wind up friends.

Doctor Sussman wasn't as easy. The phrase, "all business," never had it so good. You will remember how our first meeting went, but between that appointment and our next I learned from everyone with an opinion what a skilled doctor he is. Taking into account my own fragility during our first meeting, maybe I could have done more on my part. But it didn't get any better the next time I saw him.

Of course it didn't help that I was lying in a bed, prepped and waiting for him to perform the biopsy. He entered the room without so much as a nod and began explaining the non-invasive surgery would only take a few minutes. My wife sat next to my bed and it only takes a second to say hello so I interrupted Doctor Sussman long enough to introduce her.

"Hey, doc," I said, "This is my wife, Karen," and he did briefly pause, then, to say hi. I want to hope that all doctors and nurses under any circumstances never tune out the fact that everyone sitting and laying in those small rooms, surrounded by technical medical equipment, being probed in preparation for surgery are worried and anxious about what is happening. If ever we need comforting words from schooled professionals it is now.

After the biopsy we were scheduled to see Doctor Sussman again the following week. On that day he came into his office and immediately said hello to us both, and then it was down to business but his eye-contact and facial expressions reflected a very real and humanistic concern. He indeed seemed more cognizant of our feelings that day. He explained to me the "team" approach to cancer, briefly gave me a synopsis of what I could expect over the next few months, and once the appointment was over he told us to step into his secretary's office and line up an appointment in three months so he could check my progress. As he stood to leave I stopped him. I wanted to tell him how wonderfully I had been treated by everyone so far and to tell him how highly and unanimously revered he his among his own peers. I thought if he could hear it out loud it might swing things more favorably toward giving us a chance to proceed as two humans, not a doctor and patient. I wanted to be the difference maker Jim Kelly described, but to my own shock and surprise as I started to speak I totally fell apart and broke into tears. The weight of cancer came crashing down in front of everyone and suddenly Doctor Sussman's eyes widened and he swiftly placed a comforting hand on my shoulder, as did Karen, and I'll be darned, however strangely it came to pass, there sat three everyday humans in a doctor's office, two of them helping to calm a fallen comrade. It was a pivotal moment in my lifetime; one I will never forget.

Several days later, feeling embarrassed about my meltdown, I used my electronic connection to Guthrie Medical to send Doc Sussman a quick note:

Hi Dr. Sussman,
Jeez, sorry about that meltdown in your office. I just wanted you to know that each step

of the way so far every nurse, every doctor, every technician, and every receptionist, have not only treated me like royalty, but also to a tee have spoken very highly about you. Sometimes it's just nice to hear things like that. I also can surmise that along the way you probably wondered if all the education and years spent at it would culminate in more than a livelihood, but I can assure you, whether or not people say it out loud much, you are extraordinarily revered. That's all I was trying to convey, but the emotions of this stuff are, on occasion, getting the better of me. All of us face hurdles along our way, I've cleared my share of them, so despite the bumpy road ahead, I tread with confidence knowing you are in my corner.

Thanks, Doc. See you in October.
Roger

And in response, proving to be very much an everyday caring and thoughtful human being, Doctor Sussman replied:

Dear Roger,
The results of your PET CT shows tumor in the tongue base as previously diagnosed but no spread to elsewhere. Also, thank you for your letter. It is taking care of great people like yourself that gives fulfillment in our job. Thanks so much for your kind thoughts and I promise you, you will beat this.

Doctor Sussman's letter encouraged me as I moved onward to the next stop where I would meet the nucleus of my "team," Doctor Collier—a distinguished oncology radiation specialist, Doctor Gosain—a chemotherapy specialist, and this is also the first time I would meet Karena, whom I have already introduced. Soon into the process I would next be greeted by three radiology technicians, Mike, Charlie, and Deb, each who would routinely assume key roles in my treatments, and finally, Lauren, a registered nurse who worked alongside Karena. Every single one of these medical professionals fit the bill of difference makers.

Karena is the one who met me in the lobby and escorted me back into the radiation section where several small rooms lined the corridor. She showed me into a room to cover some preliminaries and took my vitals before exiting to go find Doctor Collier. Doctor Collier would be the one taking responsibility for interpreting my original PET CT scan and setting up a 3-D radiation computerized program specifically designed to my particular situation. After entering the room with Karena he nodded hello but got right to business by pulling up my original PET CT scan and showing me the infected area and began describing the intricate process in so many medical terms I thought to just shut up and listen for the time being. This would be no easy barrier to crack as Doctor Collier seemed a world away and on such a higher plane that maybe just this once I should leave the barrier in place. Along our way together, each Tuesday he would be running a brief checkup on me to monitor how things were going. He worked hand-in-hand with Karena and, like she had, before leaving the room that day he warned me to prepare for the worst three months of my life.

For now, I left the barrier in place. Frankly I did believe it possible that Doctor Collier somewhere among the medical terminologies had entirely lost touch with his human side. His overall brilliance seemed almost intimidating and to be honest, for once I did feel I was out of my league trying to have a meaningful conversation.

However, and I'm jumping ahead here, once treatments began it was on our very first Tuesday when Doc Collier floored me and wiped away all of my initial presumptions that I now felt asinine to have harbored. When he entered the room on that day I stood to shake his hand and exchange quick pleasantries. He seemed open to that, so as he checked my data, weight, blood pressure, and whatever else was in front of him, I asked, "How are things going for you, Doc?"

"I'm doing quite well," he replied, and I was sort of stunned by his congenial manner. Then he looked up from his notes to address

66

me more directly and continued, "But it does get hard now and then. My wife and I separated some time ago so there's always that."

"Oh, no," I answered. "It must be awfully tough with what you're expected to do for all of us to try to have a home life too."

"It is, it is," he agreed, and went back to reviewing my charts. Soon he looked up again and this time, completely out of the blue, revealed the tragedy of having lost one of his sons; worse, his son had taken his own life and the pain in Doctor Collier's face made it clear that, yes, we all have a human side, and we all have hurdles. I can't recall exact details, but his son seemingly had the best of lives working in a New York City high rise looking down each day on Fifth Avenue or The Stock Exchange, something along that order, a pillar of success at a young age. From all outward accounts Doctor Collier's son was a huge success, the epitome of what any dad would like to see their son turn out to be.

"Then one day..." uttered Doc Collier, his voice trailing helplessly and his arms opening slowly to quietly finish his sentence... "he was gone."

It was a gloomy start to be sure, but it made clear Doctor Collier did have a very human side. As the weeks passed he shared lighter moments and I came to learn how eager he is to engage so every Tuesday I would find the opportunity to ask the same question, "How are things going for you, Doc?" and I would enjoy the brighter stories. As a case in point, you would have to see Doctor Collier to fully appreciate his upcoming trip to the Bahamas. The doctor is not, repeat not, the prototype to just wing it off on a Caribbean vacation. In the first place he has fairer skin than mine, and as far as general appearance, I hope he won't be mad if I ask you to envision... well, the studious type is all that comes to mind. He's the type that would actually purchase and wear the exact wide-brimmed straw hat that he recommended for me to protect my neck area from the sun during my treatments and beyond. I'm the type that will never under any circumstances be caught under a wide-brimmed straw hat. No. I wear ball hats and sun block because I do everything in my power to hold onto the description of Toxic Masculinity. But back to Doc Collier, he indeed did intend on heading down to the hot Bahamas for a week to be with his other son and to soak up whatever he could of a relaxing week. We talked about it weekly and his excitement peaked as the date grew nearer. He hit full stride about a week prior to his trip when he talked about paddling his ass along the shores of some tiny Caribbean islands in a kayak. My jaw dropped and before I could stop myself I blurted, "You're kidding."

Even Doctor Collier laughed at my reaction and fully understood where it came from.

"No, no, I might not look the part," he said, still chuckling, "but I actually love to kayak." All I could do is stare dumbly back at him while trying to visualize it… I still can't. All I keep seeing is a wide-brimmed straw hat washing lazily ashore.

I think the vision of Doc Collier paddling a kayak is tough to beat, but he sure did come close when, after returning from the Bahamas, he turned a conversation I had initiated about ice fishing into his yearly visit to Lake George. Lake George is located far north in upstate New York and what Doc Collier seemed most hyped about was not ice fishing, but how he could not wait to see everyone "get tanked up" for the annual outhouse races across the frozen ice. You can take it from there, right? So, yes, let's not worry about Doctor Collier's human side; it is quite intact.

Doctor Collier was instrumental in saving my life. I applaud his brilliance, his wisdom, and his undying efforts. I will think of him often over whatever years I have left and be cheering for him to one day find more time for kayaks under wide-brimmed straw hats.

Back to day one of meeting my team, after my inaugural visit with Doctor Collier, Karena escorted me back out to the lobby to wait for my next appointment on the opposite side of the Cancer Center where chemotherapy and infusions take place. There I would meet the wide eyed and enthusiastic Doctor Gosain. I quickly learned to decipher Doctor Gosain's presence by the speedy rhythm of his hard-heeled shoes clicking rapidly across the laminated floors. Back in the days when I used to hire employees the very first order of business was to watch through my office window whenever an applicant showed up and parked out in the driveway. It is a far enough distance from the driveway to my front door to gather a reasonable estimate of a person's general pace. If an applicant lazily opened their door, stood gawking about, and then sauntered lethargically up toward the door their chances were pretty much squashed before our interview began. On the other hand I felt better about the applicant who stepped alertly from their vehicle and assumed a no-nonsense approach up toward the door. I still think it was one of the wisest screening methods I employed. Charging by the hour and paying by the hour, meant a person's general pace weighed heavily—I can guarantee you one thing, Doctor Gosain would have been hired before covering half the distance... which would not have taken long.

I didn't meet with Doctor Gosain much. There was just our initial meeting wherein he explained the three chemotherapy sessions scheduled and then a couple follow ups as my recovery progressed. But he remembered my face every time we did cross paths in the lobby or hallways and was always quick to the handshake, another gesture I place high marks on. Better yet, whenever Karen was with me, he smiled and nodded politely and respectfully shook her hand too. (I wonder if he's known as "old school Doc Gosain," there at the Center.)

Our initial meeting was simply to tell me to get ready for hell, but he was so pleasant about it I shrugged and said, "Let's go." We wouldn't formally meet again until the week following my final treatments. The person he saw that day was a far cry from the one he had met with in August. Despite my being a visible shambles Doctor Gosain entered the room, smiled broadly, shook Karen's hand and then mine. Next he pulled up a chair, slid it directly across from me and sat so close our knees nearly touched. He sustained deliberate and meaningful eye contact and lingered for a few long seconds before breathing a small sigh and leaning yet closer where he lowered his voice. "You have been through a lot sir, but believe me the worst is over. You have come a long, *long* way. You are going to beat this."

Doc Gosain is also the one who interpreted for us the results of my second PET CT scan upon which he reported that he and the other docs, Collier, and Sussman, were overall "very pleased." However there was still a bit of activity showing on the original infected lymph node. The hope and consensus was scar tissue from the treatments. Knowing now, though, that a future CT scan was automatically in the works Doc Gosain verified my suspicions by telling me the customary protocol would mean leaving the feeding tube in place for another six weeks.

Exasperated, I lost my filter, narrowed my eyes and said, "Shit, doc, I haven't needed to use that thing in the *past* six weeks. I hate this thing."

Sensing my frustration to be greater than he had imagined, Doctor Gosain smiled and said, "Okay, I can tell you've probably seen enough of that. Let me talk to Doctor Collier and I'll have an answer for you today or tomorrow." That very evening I was contacted by Kelly from the Center to inform me the tube could be removed in two weeks at my next appointment with Jennifer Cornish.

Perfect enough I guess.

Now Jenn. Jenn is a nurse practitioner and the instant she opens the door and enters the room you know you like her. She's quick with a big hearty smile and so easy to make laugh one wonders if she doesn't share my philosophy on barriers from the other side and tries to bust them up herself. The reason I first scheduled to see her was to monitor the PEG tube of which she is a specialist of sorts.

I treated the thing with kid gloves afraid it would pop out or malfunction in some way so immediately Jenn put me at ease by assuring me she could fix any problems right here on the spot. First, though, she needed to get her own take on the tube.

"All I need ya to do, Mr. Page, is take your shirt off and lay back on this table."

"Really?" I joked, never willing to resist such a hanging curve ball. "Then you're going to have to call me Roger unless you insist on spoiling the mood."

Still laughing she began to prod my stomach and rib cage until I called to Karen, "Jeepers Kare, get up here and watch what she's doin', will ya?"

In spite of the clowning, though, Jenn knew her stuff about these tubes and by the time we had finished I left there much more assured that the thing would be fine.

She scheduled a follow up visit to coincide with my next appointment with Doctor Sussman. The next time I saw her I'm sorry to say I had slipped far beyond the joviality of our first meeting. My voice completely shot, I was down to typing notes into my phone to let the docs read. By now, too, I was losing weight at a precarious clip and the tube no longer fit tight at all. Remembering how I felt about the person who installed it and not wanting to ever rely on him in case of an emergency I briefly described those feelings to Jenn and then typed, "You're the only one I want to help me if something goes wrong. I trust you."

Jenn read my note and was obviously touched. She sighed deeply and smiled up at me.

"Alright ya big lug," she said. "I've never done this before but I'm going to give you my cell number. I don't want you worrying about this."

I never did need to call her about the tube, but just to have the assurance someone would be compassionate enough to stand ready to help at a moment's notice made a big difference.

Finally, though, and this is jumping way ahead, there did come the big day to have the tube removed. Jenn opened the door to the small room where Karen and I waited and by this point in time all humor had been restored so in seconds we were all joking around making each other laugh and given the bantering one could easily forget why we were there. But finally Jenn got down to business.

"Alright, let's do this. Shirt off and lay on the table."

I followed along cooperatively.

Jenn then approached my side and cautioned, "Now this might hurt a bit for a couple minutes..."

"Whoa, jeepers, Jenn. You're not going to numb the area?" I fretted.

I had envisioned a couple tiny pricks of anesthesia followed by a careful incision to widen the orifice a bit in order to slide the stopper through, then a few stitches, and a gauze bandage.

"I can rub a smidge of numbing cream on there if you want but I doubt it will do much good."

"Well how are you going to take it out?"

"I'm going to have you hold down tightly onto your stomach and I'm gonna yank it outta there."

"Are you *serious*?"

"Lay down on that table and let's find out," she laughed.

"Well how 'bout a shot o' whiskey, then," I requested, "and a bullet to bite down on?"

Jenn has a wonderful laugh, and by now Karen chirped in my other ear, "Just do it, Roger, get that thing outta there."

And she was right. I had put up with the tube so long I decided to lay back and trust Jenn no matter what.

"Now you hold right down tight on your stomach," instructed Jenn, and as I did that I could feel her wrap the tube around her wrist a time or two for leverage and I thought "she's really going to *do* this…." and *wham*! Sure enough she ripped it out like an angered man starts a lawnmower and the thing made an echoing plunk like a golf ball strikes a dead oak. Shocked by the suddenness I opened my mouth to scream but nothing came out. Strangely there wasn't one iota of pain, yet there I lay with my mouth opened wide enough to shove a basketball into.

"Are you okay? Are you okay?" shouted Jenn.

I couldn't catch my breath in time to stop my voice from saying, quote: "You crazy f**ker!"

Now I'm absolute she's heard that before, but probably not from a patient. In no time she was squealing to Karen to hold the bandage, "I'm afraid I'm gonna pee my pants." But Karen was no better, crippled with laughter on my other side so I grabbed the bandage myself and from there I guess when it comes to medical pros having their human sides we'll let Jenn wear the crown.

Of course everything can't be funny and light, and when pros are at work it is no surprise they are in a different world—in my own work I was as guilty. A fellow named, Paul, worked for a colleague of mine in the landscaping world. Paul tended shrubs at a nursery run by my buddy Don and often after a hard day I would stop in and bat the breeze. Often Paul was there and we would joke and laugh about whatever we could find to joke and laugh about so Paul grew to think what a fine and funny guy I was. One time I needed some extra help on a landscaping project and asked if Don could part with Paul for the day. Don said, "Sure," Paul agreed so I lined things up for him to meet us the following morning at 8:00. Also, Paul was asked to wear long pants, not the customary shorts he wore at the nursery, and to wear good boots. Those parts he got right, but when he showed up at 8:10 he was met with an earful he'll never forget from that fine and funny guy he had been accustomed to back at the shop. As the day progressed and the job got done, Paul melded in as best he could with my regular workers and me, but by day's end he had certainly seen and heard enough. Don laughed to tell me that the first words out of Paul's mouth were, "I didn't even recognize Roger! The guy's a little intense when he works, isn't he?"

Intensity at our jobs is expected if we are to be considered worth our salt, and I agree with that. But all of us embrace at least a degree of desire to step outside of that from time to time and loosen the atmosphere up a bit.

Back to being a difference maker, it doesn't stop at cancer. It could be a relative having a bad day, a friend carping about life's struggles, a neighbor with their mower stuck in a ditch, who knows where opportunities to make a difference will crop up, but since I've started observing more closely, they do crop up more often than you might otherwise think.

As treatments began, my time for radiation was 10:30 each morning. Naturally, many of the same people were there day after day and of course gentle pleasantries eventually morphed into grander conversation as each day passed. On one such morning I struck up a conversation with an older couple when I overheard her say to him, "I'm done with this. I can't keep doing this."

The man's face showed the hurt I surmised he had felt before—surely this wasn't the first time, so I smiled and said to her, "Well you look tough as nails to me. Plus we owe it to all these incredible docs and nurses to make their investments in us pay off. We can't just quit."

She gazed back at me, not infringed at all by my interjection and grinned, "Ah, shit, I guess you're right. But for the love of god, it just gets tiring."

"That's for sure," I said, and our conversation moved quickly from there to days of old—cruise ships, lakes, golf courses, and the like, and for at least a small moment her eyes came alive and her spirit seemed revived.

When she was called for her radiation her companion looked deeply into my eyes and said, "I want to thank you for that. She needs to hear it from someone besides me."

"Hey," I said to the man, "I'm no expert, but just from what little I've been through it's easy to tell that sooner or later a person is going to say, "no more."

He nodded his head knowingly.

"If she ends up doing that, sir, it might be best not to fight it. Just stay with her and help her until the end. She's going to need you."

Again he nodded, and then he looked up with a tear trickling down his cheek and said to me, "You're a good man. You're honest."

So you see how quickly and even quietly one can become a difference maker. It really is a call to duty and along the way you will feel better, too, about yourself. Give it a try—be a difference maker for someone in need and before you know it you'll be doing it day in and day out.

The pendulum swings both ways. I had finished my treatments and had advanced into the "recovery" stage, but to tell you the truth, I did not feel as though much recovery was occurring. My coughing was still non-stop, my voice still a no-show, I was still feeding through my tube, but when an early winter snowstorm dumped on us in November I thought if I took my time I could get us shoveled out. Keep in mind shoveling snow to me means a great deal. As a seven-year-old kid it is how I earned my first income. I charged twenty-five cents a sidewalk, most of the street hired me (my mom might have had something to do with that) and as my piggy-bank bulged with quarters I could hardly wait for springtime when I could begin buying baseball cards. They were only a nickel per pack so from my winter income I could easily afford five or ten packs at a time. Each pack had five cards and a stick of gum. All of us who collected cards would now and then huddle together to trade off our "duplicates," but by exploring yet further I found I could swap a few sticks of gum for a player or two, too. I studied each player's card to the point of remembering and reciting every pitcher's ERA, strikeouts, bases on balls, and every batter's batting average, base hits, home runs, and you name it. From snowfall I developed a work ethic, business sense, and a memory that won't quit. To this day, shoveling snow is my way to pay homage, and I take it very seriously. Often sweet Karen talks about buying a snow-blower and just as often I make my plea to convince her how much that would break my heart.

So that's the frame of mind I was in as I headed out the door after the snowfall to begin digging us out.

"Please be careful, Rog," Karen sighed as I insisted on giving it a whack.

"I won't press it, don't worry," I told her. "I have all day. Don't worry," and out the door I strode.

I didn't know exactly what to expect, I hadn't exerted myself in any way at all for months. I used to be in robust shape, especially for winter activity, but one stab at the compacted snow left by the plows out by the road told me I was in too deep. Still I should do my best and see how things go. Soon, from the corner of my eye here came neighbor Joyce from three hundred yards down the hill trudging up toward me, shovel in hand. Seventy-one years old this lady is and from any distance you can feel her perpetual smile. A retired oncology nurse she never breathed a word admonishing me for my willingness to face a foot of snow, she simply asked, "Ok, where do ya need me?" Seeing the awful density out near the road she quickly suggested her husband Jim bring his backhoe up to take on the tougher stuff. She already had her phone in hand to call him. Meanwhile from the house Karen had snuck out and carved her way out to our vehicles with her little eager-beaver shovel and was working on cleaning off the vehicles and the area around them. Five minutes later neighbor Dale slowed his truck on the road and called out, "What the heck do you think you're doing? I'll be back up with my snow blower."

Oh, I got my share of shoveling in, don't worry about that, but in my condition there was no way on earth I would have made it through that dumping. But without asking a soul or saying a word, the goodness in others converged upon a sick man's driveway so swiftly it seemed overwhelming. I have felt the certain gratification that comes from helping others any number of times but nothing compares to such spontaneous generosity when you are the one who needs help.

I started the day wielding a giant shovel aiming to be the toughest guy on earth. And to be fair, I did hang in there until the snow was gone, but ultimately the toughest guy on earth huddled back indoors wrapped in a blanket, sipping hot chocolate, entirely humbled by the kindness of others.

I have spotlighted just a few of the many ways we can be difference makers. Sure, it might not change a person's life, it might be something as small as a smile while you hold a door open, but as you cultivate within yourself the desire to help others imagine if that became infectious... and then tell me it isn't. It absolutely is. You are not bound to change the world but you can change your part of the world for the time being and when others feel how it feels to be treated differently, many of them, too, will take up the chase. I guarantee it.

Prep Work And Apprehensions

After the meltdown in Doctor Sussman's office I realized no matter what type exterior you mean to portray, the truth can still break free. Willing to take Krauthammer's advice and fully accept my condition meant I was inwardly scared to death at times about what awaited. I understood from what Doctor Sussman projected that the road ahead would be foreign and often forlorn, but many of the details still seemed sketchy. At least the ball was rolling now, though, and the next step was to have a Doctor Rorabaugh install what is called a "port" into my chest. The port would be used for easy access to draw blood or to inject fluids and I would be seeing my share of each.

No need to wonder about Doctor Rorabaugh's human side, it's his professional side you might want to worry more about. I'm kidding, of course, Doctor Rorabaugh is as good as it gets. He entered the room during my pre-op appointment to get things straight and to have me sign off on the procedure.

"Gonna install a port in your chest, Mr. Page. I'm supposed to tell you it could cause blood clots, heart damage, punctured lung, seizures, and whatnot; you okay with all that?" He probably wasn't as flippant as I'm making it sound, but the way he presented it anyone could sense his disdain for the C.Y.A. part of his job. I deal with it in my own livelihood, too, so chuckled along with the doc while I signed the papers.

"Alright," he said, "How does next Tuesday morning at 9:30 work for ya?"

"Sounds good to me," I replied, and with a quick handshake I was back about my day.

On the day of the surgery Doctor Rorabaugh stepped into the pre-op room where I was being prepped for the surgery and nodded hello to Karen before he looked down at me from the foot of my bed.

"Gonna poke a hole in ya, Mr. Page," he smiled, "D'ya hunt?"

Momentarily stunned by his question it took me a minute to stammer, "Uh, yeah, as a matter of fact, I do."

"Right handed?"

"Yep."

"Okay, I'll put 'er on the left side for you."

Can you believe that? Of all the issues that could be on any doctor's mind at any time, Doc Rorabaugh thinks to ask me a very human and very important question—one even I hadn't thought of.

It was the only time I would see him, but the impression he left will last a lifetime. His concern might seem like a small thing to many people, but to a hunter, Doctor Rorabaugh is a big time difference maker.

The next step to prepare me for treatments was to have my mesh mask formed to my face. I have since heard several people marvel that after thirty-three radiation treatments I have no "burn marks." I'm wondering if this mask that was formed to cover my neck and face could be the reason. At the Cancer Center I arrived ten minutes early where a congenial voice met me the instant I made it through the doors.

"Are you Roger?" he asked.

(They have a picture of you on file these days so for medical staff to know your name before being introduced isn't that uncommon.)

"Yep, that's me," I replied, matching his smile with my own.

"I'm Mike," he said. "You're gonna get sick of me. I'm going to be one of the techs overseeing your radiation treatments."

"I won't get sick of ya, Mike," I said, shaking his hand.

"Alright, glad you're early, might as well get started. Follow me."

He escorted me into a small room where I laid flat on my back while he explained the procedure. The mesh he showed me was simply a flattened sheet at that point.

"I'm gonna soak this in pretty hot water for a minute or so and then I have to ask you to lie as still as you can while I form it over your face. It's going to be a bit uncomfortable, lots of water running down your face and neck and it might seem too warm at first but it won't be so hot as to harm you so hang tough for me if you can."

"Got it, Mike," I said.

"Are you claustrophobic?" he asked.

"Nope. I trust ya. I won't move. You go ahead and do whatever you need to."

"That's what we wanna hear," he said, and patted me knowingly on the shoulder. "It'll only take a minute."

With the moistened mesh properly heated Mike moved over to me and began pressing it into place over my face. He hadn't lied about the discomfort, but it was tolerable enough to adhere to his instructions and keep perfectly still.

"Okay," he said, finally, as he lifted the mesh and began drying my face and neck with a towel. "Wish everyone handled it that way."

"Well, Mike, to be truthful, I can see why some wouldn't. It's not exactly fun."

"No, I know it isn't," he said. "But these masks sure make the treatments go a lot better, I do know that."

From there Mike accompanied me over to the main hospital to which the Cancer Center is adjacently attached. I still needed to pass some other preliminaries like a cardiogram and EKG, things like that. Once we got those in the books we headed back to the Cancer Center where Mike showed me to the door and said, "See ya soon, my friend."

"Alright, Mike, see ya soon."

The next step, one I dreaded, was the installation of my feeding tube. As commending as I have so far been about doctors and nurses, this is one case where I won't sound so affectionate. To begin with the doctor had been on an extended vacation and on his first morning back had lined us up like cattle—something like seventeen procedures of which I was first in line. Nonetheless, without any apology he sauntered into my pre-op room a half-hour late where he ignored Karen and ignored me, too, if you want my take. He was dressed like a disco DJ, and he smelled so strong with perfume I buried my face into my blanket.

"Is this a spoof?" I wondered under my breath.

Finally he did speak, presumably to satisfy a requirement that he explain my procedure, but did so with such uninterpretable rapidity I couldn't make out a word he said. His version of English was hard to understand to begin with which isn't my fault—he should know to slow down, but what set me off the most was when he leaned over to monitor my heartbeat and lungs his cell-phone blasted off in my ear with some god-forsaken screaming ring-tone and he made no motion whatsoever to get it stopped. It takes all my resistance here to omit his name. When my tube was installed he was in such a hurry he failed to secure the clamps. In recovery when I coughed there was a sickening gurgling sound and I could feel fluid escaping slightly above my navel. Still groggy I muttered, "I think I'm leaking," but by then it was Karen who had already leaped into action to get the clamps closed properly.

"Sorry about that," laughed one of the nurses, hustling over to help Karen. But nothing about it was funny.

The tube was a game-changer. Suddenly I felt inferior, immediately a sicker and lesser man with a feeding tube protruding from my stomach. A disheartening sight, especially knowing it would be there for a long, long time.

By now we were well into August and as my treatments loomed closer I felt both anxious and scared; anxious to get fighting back, but frightened by having no idea what to expect. There finally came a day for a dry run where I was introduced to the radiation room, placed onto the bed, and when they buckled my mesh mask tightly against my face to make some target marks the harsh snapping of the restrainers sent chills down my spine. It is a sound I can hear to this day—and will forever. The mask pressed way too hard against my nose, but Mike was able to alleviate it somewhat by snipping it a bit and allowing me more air. The restraining mask locked tightly against a solid backboard and held my head rigidly in a stationary position. I closed my eyes and worked hard mentally to treat it like a wonderful nap... minus the wonderful.

The dry run completed, tomorrow would mark the beginning of treatments. Apprehensive or not, I felt ready to roll. I hadn't spoken a lot about any of the prep work on social media, most of it would seem unremarkable from a distance I suppose, but this would be a good time to update my Facebook friends.

Now it's day one of treatments. I'm sitting on the deck before sunrise and what I'm thinking mostly about is how much I long for a day down the road where I'll sit out here again waiting only to feel the sunrise while sipping rich coffee and watching my hound shift positions to plop back down with a gratified sigh. On that day I won't have an appointment for chemotherapy and what a difference it will be to have this stomach tube lying in a garbage can somewhere behind me. That alone will be a pleasant enough thought to carry a day. By then I'll know all about chemotherapy and radiation treatments and, oh yeah, the mesh mask they're going to use thirty-three times to bolt my face upright against a stiff backboard in order to hold me exactly in line with the miraculous 3-D treatments, that will be in a glorious scrap heap somewhere behind me, too.

At least that's my personal prognosis, but the truth is I am not confident at all yet about how this turns out. From what I've heard and read, I worry to death about my salivary glands, taste buds, and the like, but at least it will be nice to finally feel this swollen lymph node begin to get its head handed to it.

Maybe a year from now things really will be back on track; I'll try my best to believe it. I want to believe it. But of all the problems a patient can have, there is no cure for pragmatism. Worry about that later—I finally at least get to play the hand I'm dealt and that satisfies me enough for one day.

With the world's best doctors, technologists, nurses, and medicinal methods known to man, I am as ready as I'll ever be to get started.

Onward.

Treatments

The way it works for radiation treatments is the patient is offered to select a time from whatever is available and to be at the Center at that time every day. I chose 10:30 and would arrive fairly close to that, usually at least ten minutes early. Receptionist, Lisa, governs a small stack of plastic red cards staged each day on her desk and you must verify your birthdate in order for her to hand yours over. She sees you every day, you haven't changed a bit, yet every single day the birthdate C.Y.A. game must be covered. As I've mentioned, there came a prolonged period during and exceeding my treatment phase where I lost the ability to speak. Lisa, bless her heart, met me at the desk each day and I think I felt sorrier for her than I did me, as she had no choice but to withhold my card until I at least satisfactorily mouthed, "Five-nineteen-fifty-five." The obvious question is who on earth is going to impersonate a patient about to receive a blast of radiation?

Nonetheless, I cooperated as best I could and even if no words came out, Lisa smiled and handed me my card.

Once you secured your red card you returned to the lobby to wait for one of the techs, Mike, Charlie, or Deb, to come and escort you back into a space-aged looking, wide open room with the strangest looking contraption of a machine planted squarely in the middle. There you laid down on your back upon a narrow planed "bed" of sorts, and whatever tech was assisting today fitted your mesh mask tightly against your face and tacked it down with four bone chilling WHACK! WHACK! WHACK! WHACK's—the unforgettable sound of each restrainer echoing harshly across the room and locking your head into position.

Then everyone leaves the room.

During the first treatments it seemed haunting to feel so alone in there, but after a while you learn to trust the system. The techs monitor the treatments from an adjoining room where half the wall is a long protective glass barrier separating them from the patient.

The treatments are painless, the trick is to shut your eyes as if taking a nap. As time went by I learned to listen for certain keys to chart my progress. The machine began with a steady high-pitched whir that seemed linear to the ear, but in actuality I am sure the head of the radiation machine rotated circularly. The high-pitched whir seemed to begin at one ear, pass slowly over me, and progress to the other ear before a subtle singular CLICK, signified the end of its rotation. Each rotation took about a minute-and-a-half and in between each pass was a pause of nearly a minute before the whirring sound fired up again. Each session required only four of these rotations and always after the fourth click I presume the trio behind the glass heard a softly muttered, "Yes. Another one down," a battle cry they have probably grown accustomed to.

After the fourth rotation the door across the room immediately opened to the welcome sound of footsteps crossing the floor to my rescue. The loud snaps of the mask fasteners were just as abrasive being unfastened but in a better way. You know what I mean.

Of course along with my prescribed thirty-three blasts of radiation aimed at my throat and tongue, I was to undergo three chemotherapy sessions, one the very first day of treatments, one midway, and one toward the end. Spaced that far apart, approximately three weeks each, I should expect the heaviest doses available, but having no inkling about chemotherapy I figured it's probably better get it over with in just a few sessions than every single week... I guess.

Chemotherapy would sure come to open my naïve eyes about toughness and good attitude. In a very short time chemotherapy proved to me that you do not kick cancer's ass, as the common phrasing goes. No, cancer kicks *yours* and your objective boils down to outlasting it.

Have you ever heard of renegade country singer, Jerry Jeff Walker? Jerry Jeff was a real sort back in the day. Booze, drugs, parties, the whole nine, but, gosh, I do love his music. Once I was reading a story about Walker and I can never be sure how true or not any story about such a character could be, but I sincerely believe this one to be on the mark. Apparently Jerry Jeff had gotten too chummy with a larger man's wife and said some things you might hesitate saying even to your own wife. Well in no time things escalated to the point of Jerry Jeff winding up in a serious confrontation. Instead of apologizing and hoping for the best, the inebriated Walker sprouted off a bunch of f-bombs and then typifying the delusional oddball he could be in those days he doubled up his fists. Oh, what a dreadful error. The story goes that the large husband began punching Jerry Jeff and continued punching him until he figured he had things pretty well covered. Never to be totally defeated, though, Jerry Jeff peered up through the blood and a couple missing teeth and defiantly slurred, "Ah, y'all ain't so tough... I've had my ass kicked lots worse than this."

Well if you have never undergone chemotherapy, picture yourself as Jerry Jeff because in a lot of ways that is exactly how it leaves you. I'm not saying you can't weather the storm, but I am saying it will be one unforgettable storm.

The radiation treatments weren't tough at all at first, but as time wore on and my throat deteriorated and I needed to turn exclusively to my feeding tube to eat, and the chemotherapy wore me down, and finally my voice left the scene, it grew harder and harder to believe I would come out of this with any hope at all to ever return to a meaningful life. I'll talk more about it later, but as much as I thought I had prepared against it, depression found a way to infiltrate and the only thing on my mind was to live through the day—to survive the day.

The idea that anyone kicks cancer's ass is laughable.

I probably should not be so presumptuous in seeming to speak for all cancer patients, but when it comes to the throat I wield an amplified degree of confidence in telling you what a patient learns about good attitude, a positive approach, and fortitude. One by one, they dissipate. Trust me, if radiation is aimed at your throat, you will not have a good attitude, or a positive approach, or much fortitude left by the time it is over. Add in a few rounds of chemotherapy and the only question is how far along will you make it before you begin to lose your will.

Of course you understand that I am not advocating against a great attitude; by all means *do* have a great attitude for as long as you can sustain it, and start regaining it the instant it comes available again. But somewhere along the way don't be surprised to find it is no longer there for you. I'm just being honest.

What will be there for you is a support team that has seen it all before and knows what to expect. They know when to step in, what to do, and what to say. Trust them, they are on your side.

As my radiation treatments progressed and I totally lost my ability to speak, Mike, Deb, and Charlie, administering my treatments were sympathetic and supportive, urging me to hang tough while realizing I was slipping big time. Toward the end I existed primarily in a daze, but I don't think anyone was surprised. Radiation to the neck and throat area, according to the medical consensus, is among the very worst.

By the time I made it to my third round of chemotherapy I simply sank into the reclining chair, turned on the television for Kare, and stared at the god forsaken ceiling for four straight hours wondering why I would

97

ever be stupid enough to think this could possibly have a happy ending.

At this point, even the "pit of hell" seemed understated. I will never forget the sounds of that machine leaching poisons into my veins during chemotherapy, the shrill beeps when the fluids ran out, or the nurses counting to three before injecting the needles into my chest, and the god-awful smell of whatever that chemical is at the onset of chemotherapy. This is cancer. This is what it does to you, this is the state it leaves you in. So when outsiders talk about good attitudes, I'm going to let you in on a little secret. Cancer patients rarely talk about the things I'm talking about here, and if I were not writing about it, I wouldn't be talking about it much, either. But, yeah, there is a rock bottom and you stay mired there for a long, *long*, time.

Midway through my treatments, particularly after my voice betrayed me, I could feel the descent worsening. I am sure my Facebook update carried a more demoralizing tone than most friends of mine are accustomed to hearing from me, but I went ahead anyway:

Well the ship has sure hit the sand. Today is my second chemo treatment meaning I'm nearly half-way through. This one is going to floor me big time but I would hope to be more prepared than I was on the first one which ambushed me to a point where I have never felt so beaten.

I don't count the days anymore, had to go robotic; do what you're supposed to and don't break down. The radiation has devastated my throat, food tastes like burned rubber, swallowing ignites piercing pain from ear to ear, so except for some swallows of water here and there the throat is closed until further notice. That being the case, this PEG tube and I went straight from hate to best buddies— yeah—once I quit pouting I have actually become quite proficient with the thing—might even make a You-Tube video! That is as close as I can get to joking right now.

Sleep comes in two hour cycles (if I'm lucky) and for a tough guy I sure seem moved to tears a lot, mostly when I move over to pet Audrey at 2:30 AM and although she would have no way to understand why our world so suddenly stalled, her tail thumps happily for at least the moment. And when I think of all the added burdens piled upon Karen and how she stands tall in the face of it all... more tears. So as far as being a tough guy goes, I'm trading that in for just knowing on the other side of this how happy I will be to simply resume being the husband and companion they rely upon. For now, though, I have deteriorated exactly as my doctors and nurses predicted. Nobody lied.

BUT

Nobody is EVER GOING TO SEE IT, either. Those nurses, docs and radiologists that are saving my life might as well think I'm just the biggest jolly bundle of joy they've ever dealt with. And when it comes to FB, except for these occasional updates wherein I promised to be honest, all you guys are going to see are these big ol' horse-teeth of mine smiling away while I post too many pics of my dopey hound. I know I can count on you to just go with it. I despise doom and gloom even as I wallow through it, but I continue to feed off the encouragement and optimism that many of you have kept me armed with during this battle.

Ultimately I won't make it to the end of this on my own like I said I could. It takes more than a good attitude—lots of good attitudes have succumbed to cancer. It takes more than a tough guy, too. At the end of this, Karen, Audrey, Dr. Collier, nurses Karena and Lauren, and radiologists Mike, Charlie, and Deb will be dragging me across the finish line... just like everyone said it would happen. And I'm okay with that. I think they all know I have done my best to keep my demeanor above the pain for as long as I can, and if the shoe was on the other foot they all know I would be equally committed on their behalf. I promised to make their investments in me worth it and they promised to get me across the finish line. So as battered and wrecked as I feel right now, it is balanced by knowing at the same time, I have never in my life felt more loved.

Life At Home

Ever since discovering the lump, and suspecting its ramifications, my life had begun to change. Even at the onset when it was just an earache there were times when my ear hurt badly enough that I needed a heating pad. Throughout three decades of rigorous work and non-stop wintertime activity I had never in my life thought of using or needing a heating pad... for anything. Swallowing became tougher and tougher, or so I thought. Compared to what lay in store, I would end up longing to be able to swallow like I could back then. Ultimately, when swallowing does again become automatically doable I will never in my life take it for granted. It is awfully debilitating when each swallow hurts ear to ear and even gets worse as treatments proceed.

And prior to the lump, much of my life was spent out of doors where my activity level would best be described as constant; never a dull moment. That changed in a heartbreaking way and the instant my treatment schedule was laid out before me it simplified what had lurked as a challenging decision—do I try to continue working. My work has been drastically reduced for semi-retirement, I treat lawns is all. I apply fertilizers, organics, lime, insecticides, and I also spray herbicides for broadleaf weed control. But once my tube had been installed, and facing thirty-three radiation treatments along with three chemotherapy treatments, the writing was on the wall. I felt confident I could count on most of my customers, many of which have been with me for so long we've become friends. Nonetheless, I felt a bit nervous in sending them the news in a letter and hoping for the best.

I worded it as best I could, crossed my fingers, and sent the letters out.

Dear (Customer)

Many of you are already aware I have been diagnosed with carcinoma at the left tongue base and an adjacent lymph node, set off by a virus called HPV, something that can nowadays be vaccinated against. After meeting with a highly motivated, highly skilled, and highly optimistic treatment team last Friday I now have a more concrete vision of what to expect over the coming months. A port for chemotherapy treatments has been installed along with a feeding tube (eating will wind up difficult during the process), and I will be outfitted with a mesh mask to be worn for radiation treatments. There will be 33 radiation treatments in conjunction with 3 five-hour chemotherapy sessions.

I trust you to understand what I want to ask of you. I am determined to invest one-hundred percent commitment to fortify the efforts of this incredible group of medical professionals promising to get me through this. To do that, I feel it necessary to postpone my work during this fight, so I guess the best way to say it is I'm asking you to be on my team, too.

The prognosis yields every reason to believe I will be in shape to resume next spring. I hope to contact you in early March with an annual contract as in years past. If it somehow goes the other way I will be first in line to help you find a replacement. My doctors are unanimous in the belief I will emerge well. A PET CT scan verifies no other cancer besides that localized in the neck area, the treatment methods of 3D radiation is so incredibly precise, the expertise of the medical personnel so focused, and my own resolve so positive, that I have every reason to consider my livelihood—a livelihood I indeed cherish, to be simply on momentary hold.

As far as lawns go, applications omitted this fall should not make a discernible difference and I can catch us back up on weed infestations and pH sustainability in one application next springtime. Additionally the lawns won't suffer much from a temporary void of nitrogen which can be caught up quickly as well. Aside from unattended weeds this fall, in most cases the lawns are in pretty decent shape.

If you do decide to make a change I completely understand, but if you decide to bear with me I owe you an eternal debt of gratitude. The doctors have warned me that in order to get to the other side of this I am about to enter the worst two to three months of my lifetime. In return I have promised to go to whatever lengths are demanded to make certain their investments in me pay off.

I WILL GET THERE.

Thank you for hearing me out, and I ask that you please respond to this letter so I can be assured everyone has been made aware of the situation. Most of all, thank you for letting me include you on my team as I fight this.

Yours,
Roger

In no time at all, just like my Facebook friends had done, my customers, with a stunning outpouring of support eliminated any lingering apprehensions. When quarterback Jim Kelly spoke about difference makers, I am beginning to believe most humans are already onboard.

The next toughest hurdle was the fact I would not be deer hunting this season. For those who don't hunt, you might not think much about it, but to a man who has spent over forty seasons out in the woods, and not only when deer are in season, it loomed as a crushing blow. During the coming months deer season would plainly yield to the priority of saving my life. I would sacrifice this hunting season in hopes to envision many seasons yet down the road. With my perspective in order I grit my teeth and came to grips with it.

And out ahead of deer season, say from late August until opening day October first, it is the very best time of year for Audrey and me to spend time together out in the woods. She is a constant companion out there "helping" dad construct new ground blinds or clearing shooting lanes out in front of our tree stands, all of that stuff. Instead, the two new stands neighbor Mike helped me put up a while back sat vacated. With any luck, next season Audrey and I will get back out to those stands and get things squared away. But this season Audrey and I stayed home while the new stands sat abandoned. I should probably quit talking about it.

It didn't take long once treatments began for me to notice changes. After seven treatments Karen and I were able to make it to a friend's sixtieth birthday party where there was an impressive spread of food, including chicken and macaroni salad, two of my favorites but I could tell things weren't right. I ate the salad and most of the chicken, but the following weekend when I wanted one last stab at chicken wings they tasted so strange I couldn't eat them. That was about the end of conventional eating for me and with some reluctance I turned to my feeding tube and began feeding mostly on a product called, "Boost." I guess you would call it a beefed up milk product, full of vitamins, protein, and all that jazz... you can tell I wasn't thrilled.

I had previously been warned the taste of food would be affected by both, chemotherapy, but especially the radiation promising to zap my salivary glands into oblivion. So I knew the score, but now that it was actually here and happening I realized it would be months before I would eat food again in any way resembling the conventional manner; it added mightily to the sinking feeling that had already begun. For the duration of my treatments and beyond I would be eating and doing most of my drinking, too, through a tube protruding from my stomach.

By now the kitchen table had taken on the look of a mini-pharmacy, prescription pills for nausea, post chemotherapy pills, dissolvable nausea pills, and little by little the strange assortment grew. Many or most of the prescriptions did no good, at least in my rebellious eyes, so those I silently sidestepped and left alone. Before cancer, I took a tiny aspirin and a vitamin E each morning. Because I had let my weight balloon recently I had been put on a light blood pressure pill, too, so I did take one of those now and then. The nausea pills weren't really optional, especially the ones prescribed as part of the chemotherapy process so I went ahead and took those. Swallowing had by now become nearly impossible so I crushed whatever pills I was willing to take and poured them through my feeding tube.

And then there was the constant coughing. My god, the coughing once it got started seemed relentless. I couldn't sleep because of it and had to learn the oddest tricks to curtail what I could of it. I learned after "eating" that I needed to sit high up so I stacked the couch with pillows and when even that didn't seem sufficient I went to the basement and retrieved my boat cushions and brought those up to be part of the living room décor for the next few months. I learned that if I leaned way forward and bowed my head low the coughing would subside quite substantially. Great discovery, but once I tried any other posture the coughing returned. To sleep I did discover another trick was to essentially starve the throat of water. By doing that I guess I cheated the throat of anything to cough, but however it worked, I could at least fall asleep for an hour or two deep into the morning. Lying down, however, was out of the question. Not only did the coughing begin immediately but lying down ignited dry-heaves almost instantaneously. Dry-heaves became such a routine part of life I didn't even hustle to the sink any longer. Just made my way out there and spent the next three minutes going into the most violent convulsions known to man. I swear my stomach was trying to invert itself and this went on a half-dozen times a day at its peak. I surmise it due to all these foreign medications I was flirting with that I suddenly realized the onset of edema had inflated my ankles and feet like a parade float. The swelling ended up consuming my calves as well and got so bad it could qualify as a deformity if you ask me. Lower and lower I sank.

What were they *doing* to me?

The radiation treatments were painless but the culmination made me wonder how much of my throat needed to be torn to shreds to beat this crap. My guess was all of it. At the time of my second chemotherapy treatment my throat had essentially become functionless.

The chemotherapy was painless too, I guess, but you knew in two to three days the pain would sure show up. Maybe not in an acute way, but the sickness and the weakness, the nausea and the discomfort were constant and relentless. If this is a cure, I cannot imagine the intensity of the disease.

I had agreed to invest my trust in a medicinal world of which I know nothing. I respected my doctors and nurses immensely, but I could feel myself sinking deeper and deeper into my own seclusion where I would silently deal with this on my own terms—depression.

Karen, as you would expect, wisely knew to refrain from artificial encouragement—she could plainly see and hear what I was going through so trying to soothe me in some way would only seem frivolous. Instead, she did her best to keep me comfortable, a soft backrub now and then, a friendly pat on the shoulder, things like that, but she didn't try, even with good intentions, to prod me in any way. I'm sure the volume on the television was nearly inaudible for her, and of course I couldn't speak so our only communication occurred through our eyes and gestures, but we made it work. Time ticked differently for both of us; she still worked on a schedule albeit flexible enough to accommodate for driving me to my appointment each day. But the minute we returned home she took off for her work day where she worked from noon until six o'clock and then made up the balance of her hours on the weekends. She

never uttered one word of complaint about it—
I knew she wouldn't. Meanwhile, once we
returned home each morning and Kare left for
work, I turned out the lights, sat in the same
place on the couch, buried myself in blankets,
closed my eyes, and fought the constant
coughing. The television remote lay idle, my
wireless headphones remained fully charged
but untouched, e-books I had downloaded
failed to lure me in, and Audrey lay across the
way offering an occasional sigh, trying to
understand this unfamiliar demeanor. Her
eyes conveyed a sadness that I felt helpless to
address.

Would it all work out?

I began to wonder.

I would have far preferred to be angry. I
would relish feeling sorry for myself and
moaning about how unfair this is. I wouldn't
even mind bursting into tears. Those things
are at least indicative of a pulse. Currently, I
sat still in the same place on the couch,
coughing and waiting for time to pass. It
seemed hard to imagine a way back up from
this far down.

The Pit Of Hell—Depression

I almost think it advisable to pause for a moment to apologize for the somber, even desperate tone, lately, but this is the cancer I signed up to tell you about. I promise you before we are done we will evolve to higher ground, but for now, like it was when I was going through it, there is no immediate relief.

I am not a psychology expert although I did major in it for a while in college and did retain enough to incorporate it into the positive aspects of my life, particularly my working life in dealing with employees, retailers, customers, and you name it. A background in psychology can be of some value, but could I really detect depression? I think so. Having become a well-grounded person in my age, always thinking positively, always striving to do better, always active and ambitious, it seems impossible, unless for depression, for that type person to allow themselves to tumble this far down.

But this is the second time for me.

My first visit came after a month long vigil in helping our finest hound ever, Daisy, through her final month of life. Only eight years old, the nasal malignancy that attacked her was the most vicious opponent I had ever faced until now. I stayed strong for her, nursed her through the days, kept her at my side, slept at her side, and on her last day, made sure her last breath was taken while being held firmly in my arms. I loved that hound so much—she is the only dog that ever understood me back, and I feel good for any of you who know what I am talking about. I love all our dogs, of course, but Daisy was different and there will always be a piece of my heart that I will never get back. And I'm okay with that. The instant she was gone and no longer needed me, I caved to a darkness of which I had never before experienced and not for one instant did I try to fight it. If ever a companion was worth every tear.

It lasted the better part of a week. I knew what was happening far surpassed ordinary or expected grieving, but I knew, too, I would make it past it. Frankly it seemed quite right to let it run its course. I know how that must sound, but in that case depression seemed to fit like a glove.

If a person can inwardly be confident of making it through to the other side of depression, no matter how tough the struggle gets, I'd say let it run its course. I'm obviously no doctor, but twice now I have ridden the coattails of depression across the worst times of my life and in each case found it to pose as an anesthesia of sorts.

(*Please don't think I am confusing my acute situations with chronic depression, I understand the difference and would never condone letting chronic depression simply run its course; in doing my own C.Y.A. I thought it best to mention that.*)

In this most recent case depression ran beyond a couple weeks and at its worst I needed to check into the Emergency Room, something I had never in my lifetime done. The coughing was so disruptive and so convulsive that I worried there might be other things happening to me. But after most of a full morning in the E.R. they discharged me without finding anything much out of alignment with a cancer patient toward the end of treatments, of which I needed to make it through one more week. If you had asked me six or seven weeks back to imagine how it would feel to have twenty-eight out of thirty-three in the bag I would have longed for this day, but right now all I could ask of each day is that it come and go. Worse, my final chemotherapy treatment was on the Tuesday of the final week. By now I was no longer posting on Facebook, in fact I wasn't responding to emails or messages, so the only world existing was an inner form of survival wherein all that mattered was to make it to the end. The dry-heaves were at their worst, the coughing was constant, and by now I had to carry a cup around with me full time in which to spit. I don't understand salivary glands for beans, but my throat continuously filled with phlegm and each cough brought it up. Swallowing hurt so badly that the best recourse was to keep a cup handy and over time the routine seemed sickening, but fit right in.

I wanted to lay down so badly that one morning I went into the bedroom to lay on the bed just to feel what laying down felt like again. I lasted about a minute before being overwhelmed by acute dry-heaves, but the laying down part felt so good I went back after the dry-heaves subsided and did it again. This time I lay there coughing for a good three minutes, but if felt like a fair enough trade, just to remember what laying down felt like. I would return to that practice a few times over the next days, but sleeping that way was out of the question.

To be honest, I recall very little about my final week of treatments. Having no voice with which to communicate, each time coming out of radiation I would nod at Karena and mouth the words, "I'm trying, Karena, I'm trying," and one day close to Friday she finally called across the room, "Almost there, Roger. You're gonna make it."

Tuesday was chemotherapy day and like I said earlier, I slouched in the recliner, handed the television remote to Karen and then stared at the rotten ceiling for the next several hours. I hated this place, I hated this machine, and I hated that I had plummeted so far down into the pit of hell that I seemed to no longer recognize these are the very things saving my life.

With Tuesday's chemotherapy my weekly "how's it going" appointment with Doctor Collier was pushed back to Wednesday. I know he knew immediately I was barely hanging on. I surely wouldn't be interested in the Bahamas or Lake George today so he briefly examined me, checked my mouth, studied my vitals, and said, "Listen here, my friend. I know you're at the end of your rope but things are looking really good. You're holding up incredibly well."

I felt a tear begin as I looked this man in the eye and cursed myself for ever once doubting his human side. He knew exactly what I needed to hear—whether or not either of us believed a word of it. He is brilliant in more ways than one. It was just a solo tear that etched its way down my face, but it was the first I had cared to shed in weeks. Maybe things would be okay after all.

Two more days of treatments came and went and on my final day Charlie the radiation tech unbolted my mask and asked if I wanted to keep it.

I shook my head vehemently and the sour look on my face conveyed the inward feelings I couldn't say aloud, but Charlie sure understood them. "Not a chance, Charlie. Throw that piece of shit right out there in the Chemung river so nobody ever has to see that piece of shit again," and I meant every last word.

After he tossed my mask aside, I shook Charlie's hand and mouthed how much I appreciated his help through all of this. Usually Karena sat at her desk on my way out from radiation, but not today—I would have at least wanted her see me physically walk out that door for the last time. Doc Collier wasn't anywhere to be seen, either, so I made my way unceremoniously to the main lobby where Karen waited anxiously.

I had at one time imagined the magical celebration that must surely occur following the final treatment but this was nothing of the sort. Minus any fanfare whatsoever I shuffled out the doors is all. Karen stayed close and ready to steady my arm if need be but on our way across the parking lot she said, "You made it, Rog," and although she couldn't muster much of a celebratory tone, either, the words were good to hear. The truth is we both

117

knew I was hanging by a thread—Kare, too, understood depression had a foothold.

In a strange twist, however, recalling my trip last Friday to the E.R., a trip I probably never needed to make, the doctor there prescribed a cough suppressor with codeine. It became one of the few prescriptions I did latch onto, although it is considered a narcotic. As I worked with the codeine I had recently found by taking two doses, one around six or seven o'clock in the evening and another between ten and eleven o'clock that night I could count on the phlegm drying up enough so that I could gain some pretty decent sleep. By mid-week following my final treatments, the chemotherapy slowly wearing off, and the codeine helping me sleep, I began to sense a bit of relief from the listlessness that had me feeling almost comatose at times. Not a major breakthrough by any means, I was still in a bad way, but I did sense hope on the horizon.

Footnote—The Bell

When you finish your treatments there is a bell to ring. You have probably heard about it. On day one of my treatments I longed for a day coming when I would ring that bell. I envisioned Karen videoing the moment so I could share my huge victory on social media and then we could break out the balloons and party horns. Back then I had no idea that any form of frolicking or celebration would seem so out of place because back then there was only me and there was only my case of cancer to consume my thoughts. But as days passed and other's faces became familiar I learned either from directly speaking with them or overhearing enough about them that here was a revolving door of human beings that were at one time living vibrant lives with common desires but were now traveling on the wings of fear, doubt and hope—just like me. It grew to be a sobering lobby, a place to grow up fast.

My particular case had a decent prognosis for recovery. The HPV virus is noted for containment and beyond that my original PET CT scan verified nothing else of concern. It was easy at first for me to bop about the lobby upbeat and smiling, helping others load and unload at their car doors, trying in earnest to be a diligent difference maker. I learned the names of all of the staff and some of my fellow patients, right down to the happiest girl on earth, a custodian named, Tammy, but we called each other "Smiley," to give you a flavor. Of course as my own treatments went along and robbed me of my voice, and finally pitched me into this pit of hell both Karena and Doctor Collier had spoken of, I wasn't so inclined to run for mayor anymore; toward the end it was all I could do to make it through the door toting my spit cup and slouching in a seat waiting for Charlie, Mike, or Deb to come and escort me back into the radiation room for today's session.

Not once during my seven weeks of daily visits to the Corning Cancer Center did I hear that bell ring. Not once. And now I know why. An individual among others with varying plights grows less selfish by the day. Remember the lady and the man I talked about earlier, the ones where the lady said she'd had enough? When you are talking eyeball to eyeball with that person, those people, you are talking with someone very aware this will probably not end well for them; yet tooth and nail they are fighting back because fighting back is the only semblance of purpose they have left. It is not the same conversation people enjoy at the grocery store. When you consider such fear, such honesty, and such bravery and then multiply it by every single person that walks through those doors, it becomes clear as a bell why this one never rings.

A Slow But Steady Revival

Nobody lied.

The pit of hell is a very real place and if you are ever diagnosed with cancer your objective will be to make it to the other side knowing there is no way around it. Lucky for us all, there are medical pros and medicinal technology to guide us through. That seems so benign here in writing, but in real time, it is these proficient experts and the incredible tools at their disposal that will carry you should you begin to fail. They have seen a million patients like me, bright outlook, great attitude, ready to beat whatever odds, and although all of that is good, the pros realize all good things will dissipate and are prepared for it.

I find it hard to believe that my story is much different than anyone who has endured radiation in the throat area. According to everyone I have talked to, it is the very worst situation—ruined taste buds, wrecked salivary glands, uncontrollable phlegm, and a throat perpetually "exponentially sorer than you have ever experienced before," is how NP Sandra Brewer told it.

Nonetheless I would prefer a plight with at least a hopeful prognosis than I would one less forgiving in which the writing is on the wall. Those patients facing the realization of a certain outcome must test their bravery in ways unimaginable. I would stop short of calling myself lucky by any means, but it could have been worse.

For those with a prognosis suggesting the chance to go on to live many more years, it must often come accompanied by the sobering caveat that we first traverse the pit of hell. As I've mentioned, the first time I heard the phrase was by Karena and soon after, Doctor Collier echoed it; two who have seen it enough, albeit from the outside looking in. I learned to call it that, too, and so will anyone else who ends up knowing it firsthand. I have a friend, Brian, constantly dealing with weekly dialysis, who likes to say, "God doesn't deal us anything we're not strong enough to handle," or something along those lines. That seems a fine rhetorical way to describe making it across to the "other side" where we should be able to pick ourselves up and at least begin to claw our way out.

After I made it past my final treatment I surmised that in time I would be regaining enough awareness and gumption to begin my slow trek up the other side. But it wouldn't happen right away. Each evening when Karen came home we did watch television but I suspect the volume was low enough to bug her to no end. Finally on a Thursday night a full week following my final treatment I tuned into the football game and watched with enough interest that I was able to turn the volume up to an interpretable level. That was a good sign. By the following Sunday the full slate of NFL games found me interested enough to want to offer my astute input to coaches and referees. Of course it is true they couldn't hear me, never have, but today the odds were even worse as my voice wasn't yet back in play. Still, I could feel the beginning of a pulse and when that afternoon I randomly rose to my feet and donned my sweatshirt and boots to take Audrey outside for a brief walk I could feel a strengthening breath chipping away, trying like the dickens to break through.

Another week passed and slowly but surely I seemed to grow more alert. Each morning I awoke a bit earlier than the last, and each time I took Audrey outside to fetch the mail and newspaper we would linger a bit longer for her to clown around. The increasing smiles she brought suggested my breakout loomed nearer and nearer.

One morning I woke up and headed to the kitchen where it was customary to start the day by pouring a Boost through my feeding tube. Next, I would sit elevated on my spot on the couch to let the Boost settle in my stomach, but today for some reason I walked past my spot on the couch and instead moved curiously toward my office where I hadn't opened the blinds or turned a light on in over a month. At the door I turned on the lights before moving across the room to twist open the blinds. I paused, then, for a long moment to take in the mounted deer, two bears, all the fish, my magazine articles displayed on the near wall, scattered pictures of a life that had been going so well, and finally I pulled my chair from beneath the desk, sat at my computer, and brought up the abandoned manuscript to my landscaping book. Perhaps still too fragile to actually compose anything, I read some of it over and next decided to take a look at a couple of the videos Karen and I had prepared for You-Tube to coordinate with the book. The title of the book is, *The Landscape Tamed*, and last spring and summer Kare and I had filmed thirteen videos to go along with the writing. As the current video progressed, the old me energetically bounced around animatedly declaring how gol-darned important it is to learn about this pruning. My arms flailed back and forth as I pleaded with viewers to learn how to *do* this. I jumped from shrub to shrub with the vigor of a teenager and my voice boomed with enthusiasm. I looked healthy, I sounded vibrant, my pace seemed infectious, and although I missed that person dearly, I realized as the video played that he was still here—still fighting—still alive. When the video finished playing I turned to my keyboard and began typing for the first time in eons. In next to no time the keyboard thumped rapidly to accommodate my fingers pumping out an eruption of pent up words that came spilling forth to mark another of those pivotal moments in my lifetime I shall never forget.

As the next days passed, fueled by renewed efforts toward the book, I happily discovered other norms beginning to fall back into place. Football and hockey on television were games now not to be missed, especially one significant Monday night game when our beloved Seahawks took the field. Don't mess with the Seahawks on Monday Night Football, and this was no exception. Triggered by an exceptional touchdown catch, I meant to mouth, "Our Seahawks are on fire!" and the word "fire," rang out so sharply that both Karen and I jumped back wide-eyed and startled. When I slowed down and concentrated, I repeated, "our Seahawks are on fire," and every single word was audible! It wasn't pretty by any means, but entirely interpretable. Ear-to-ear smiles split both our

125

faces and as badly as I yearned for a third go I knew not to push my luck; it hurt to force the words out the second time. But, hey, call me a true fan, man. Leave it to my status as a Seahawk "Twelfth Man"—our full-throat volume being so disruptive to our opponents—to be paramount in my voice promising to return.

With each passing day, too, Audrey seemed to sense an evolving revival. To be painfully honest I had not been much of a "dad" these past couple months but now that I was spending more time with her outdoors to get the mail or just to get some air she sensed the ol' man might be pulling through after all. One morning she arrived at my office doorway clutching a tennis ball in her teeth and her eyes seemed to beg hopefully that maybe today we could resume playing ball again for the first time in months. Seeing her that way brought instant tears, but shit I was becoming so used to those I didn't even fight them anymore. I rallied enough to hone my gaze and when I clapped my hands loudly to convey, "Gimme that ball right now!" my aggressive mannerisms ignited her to charge forth with mock growling that has never before seemed so convincing. She kept it very clear that my chances at that ball were zero to none as she snarled and danced gleefully about the floor. I have never seen her eyes so full of outright delight, and maybe mine, too.

Things were looking up.

My work on, *The Landscape Tamed,* blossomed into a full-blown manuscript ready for editing and in between edits, I began this book. Still mostly house bound my muscles presumably continued to sag but my fingers were flying on the keyboard and my mind was in constant motion.

Sooner or later a mind in constant motion is going to begin wondering when eating again might be possible. I hadn't even tried. My original thoughts were to try soft foods, cottage cheese, pudding, soups, things like that. Sandy Brewer had suggested mashed potatoes soaked in butter and that sounded pretty good. What a strange feeling, to sit down with a spoon and a tiny cupful of potatoes. I tentatively brought the potatoes to my mouth and the foreign feel of food caused my lips to curl in discomfort and I couldn't chew very well it seemed, although what's to chew. I was nearly afraid to swallow; I wasn't even sure how wide my throat might open to allow food down. When I did swallow the potatoes I could somewhat taste them and it was familiar enough so that I stood my ground at the table while Karen silently cheered for me to finish them off. It took a while but at last I made it through, mostly to say I had done it. As far as eating goes, it was at least a start.

Each day I might try something new and during the first trials most of them failed. Either I couldn't chew properly yet, or I couldn't ascertain a predictable taste, but if either case prevailed I would reject the food.

Liquids were a happier story. The instant I decided to try drinking orally rather than relying on the tube, things went well. All of the liquids I had previously consumed via my tube proved to be easy enough to swallow that I could start using my throat again on a fairly consistent basis. There was a low point during my treatments where I had to be warned by Karena, Lauren, and Doctor Collier to at least try swallowing on an hourly basis. Each morning any of the three who saw me would ask if I was swallowing at least liquids and most of the time I wasn't lying when I nodded affirmatively. But the pain was simply excruciating. Still, I had to weigh that against the stern warnings from all three that there is a realistic chance for one to lose the ability to swallow altogether and having to relearn it would necessitate rigorous rehab. For a spell before their persistent warnings it hurt so badly to swallow I had completely abandoned the practice. So it loomed as a big moment when I realized I had at least progressed to a point where I could now bypass my tube in order to swallow liquids. You can imagine, too, how I breathed more easily to know my involuntary swallowing muscles had retained their memory so all's well on that front. I was pleasantly surprised, too, to find the taste of liquids to be entirely predictable. What a special treat that first gulp of V-8 juice turned out to be. I felt myself sigh deeply and after finishing my first small six-ounce can, I poured another. In no time I texted Karen to suggest stepping up to quart sized bottles of V-8 instead of buying these little sissified six-ounce cans. After cautiously avoiding any addiction whatsoever to prescriptions and narcotics, I'm afraid the same cannot be said for V-8 juice. During my last checkup Sandra needed me to up the ante on electrolytes to get my potassium, calcium, and sodium back in the game so I had begun to consume more Gator-Aid, fruit juices and nectars through my tube. But now, transitioning to drinking orally, I was happy to discover that every flavor of Gator-Aid, fruit juices, and nectars, tasted as expected. With my throat completely operable for fluids I decided to try some hot chocolate and my eyes ballooned as it eased down my throat. The warmth soothed my throat even better than the nectars but more importantly my wheels began turning toward the next logical step. Do you suppose coffee might be doable? What if I could experience the deep rich taste of strong black coffee again? After months and months, I brewed some coffee and poured a cupful. I waited for it to cool a bit. I could smell the rich aroma and that alone gave me high hopes. When I decided it was time to roll I took a tentative sip of the black coffee. Immediately my palate erupted to welcome an old faithful friend and the taste lingered long after I swallowed the coffee down. Of all the little victories that would eventually add up to recovery, this would be hard to beat.

On the heels of my successful new drinking program came my first true eating victory. Most of what I had tried was based on food texture being soft and pliable but none of that was working well. Maybe a different angle would be better. It seemed to me that everything I had tried had no familiar taste and none of it broke down well due to lack of saliva I guess. A mouthful of mashed potatoes stayed a mouthful of mashed potatoes for a full minute and probably would have stuck there all day had I not figured to swallow sooner or later. It all went down, but not like I had imagined it should. Instead of soups or soft foods, why not try something with more structure that could be chewed effectively and might turn out easier to swallow than the softer foods that were not breaking down. I knew the perfect thing to try. What if I could eat a venison hotdog? It seemed to me some meats might be doable so I thawed a hotdog and fried it. When it was done I cut it into tiny slices, let it cool, and took the plunge. The instant the hotdog touched my tongue I could taste every last bit of it, I chewed it well enough to safely swallow and probed my fork toward another slice. I had some mouth sores lingering yet, particularly on the lower tongue that had been directly targeted during radiation. The salt from the hotdog did irritate that area a bit, but all in all I ate it with enough comfort to call it a success.

By now, too, I had resumed communications with the outside world, so could hardly wait to announce on Facebook:

"I just want to state two things loudly and clearly—I can drink coffee and eat venison hotdogs again!"

Of all the more intricate messages I had posted, this was mostly tongue in cheek, yet the happy responses flooded in by the dozens. It's the little things, I guess.

From that point, eating became experimental based primarily on curiosity. Things I had so badly yearned to taste again now seemed at least possible so let's get started. Of course right away I wanted sugar. To my dismay all things sugar were tasteless. Karen baked a pumpkin pie for Thanksgiving which was nearly here and a couple days early I snuck a slice. Anxiously I doused a giant load of whipped cream upon my prize and cut a small piece and shoved it into my mouth... nothing... zero... can't taste a thing... sucks.

Frustrated by that I asked that she bring home a small little cup of ice cream for me to try. Maybe a mocha-coffee type thing would rally up some flavor. I opened my ice cream and let it soften a bit before I swirled my spoon across the top and loaded it up for the next trial... nothing... zero. Obviously sweets were not back in the strike zone yet, but just to be sure I asked Karen to whip up the most ridiculously sugar-suicide treat imaginable, our fake peanut butter fudge made quickly from peanut butter, powdered sugar, and loads of butter. When that registered another rotten zero on the taste buds I thought to sink back into woeful depression... but then quickly remembered I have coffee and hotdogs.

Thanksgiving came and we knew far in advance not to grab a giant turkey like usual. There are only two of us, but each year Karen likes to bake a pretty sizeable bird. This year we knew better so she purchased a finer cut of turkey breast, made stuffing which I had a lot of confidence in, and some mixed vegetables and gravy. I was able to eat a small portion of each, but the stuffing in particular went down pretty well so I concentrated on that.

To be honest, all of this eating is only worth celebrating when you compare it with feeding through a tube. It still was very hard to swallow, the mouth sores still reacted painfully to anything salty or spicy, and chewing wasn't quite a lost art, but it needed to be relearned in the sense of using the entire mouth with confidence rather than chewing just tiny particles. For now, I was not chewing and swallowing with total confidence, but little by little things were leaning in a positive direction.

What I began to crave, and not surprisingly, was a green salad. After months of Boost my poor stomach must be yearning for some healthy roughage but currently there had been a scare on romaine lettuce causing salmonella forcing a recall so our local stores weren't stocked. Best wait a week. When Karen at last did bring a bag of prepared salad home the next challenge wound up being to find a dressing that would work. Surprisingly thousand island, my usual favorite, tasted tart and foreign, as did honey mustard and ranch. Finally we hit home with blue cheese. Deviled eggs long ago passed the test so I could make a nice salad with lettuce, boiled eggs, and blue cheese dressing. It worked. To be able to eat salad again wasn't quite the victory of coffee and venison hotdogs, but right up there, anyway.

And any diligent eater knows it wouldn't take long for pizza to crack the radar. Karen took a Friday off to cart me to two doctors' appointments and on the way home we stopped at a local favorite pizzeria called Aneillo's. They pump out some fantastic thin crust pizza and I felt sure I could get a piece down. Instead of our usual large, Kare ordered a medium and we came home with our pizza. Once in the door I ripped open the box and raced to the living room with my piece of pizza and dove in. It worked. A bit of discomfort in the lower mouth but by the time the carnage was done I had knocked out three slices of Aneillo's pizza.

Although I couldn't call it the joy it once was, evident by phrasing it "doable," eating seemed a part of a necessary climb back to the top of the other side. How long it will take to resume eating as the ultimate joy it once was, who knows, but it seems quite probable that the day will come... that's good enough for me at this point.

I don't recall a defining moment, but eventually it came to pass that I needn't carry my spit cup around with me any longer. I don't want to be graphic about it, but the saliva now was of a different sort, not nearly as intrusive or prolific so it naturally went down on its own. Along with that, the constant coughing had subsided. I still had awful coughing fits at times, but they were sporadic and sometimes several hours might pass without a fit. Dry-heaves long ago left the scene so it all added up that it was high time to test the waters in lying down. Of all the victories to be had, this one could prove the ultimate. I stretched my legs out onto the couch and curled up into a comfortable fetal position and waited for the coughs to kick in. Nearly a full hour later I awoke with a start, but there I laid stretched right to the max. Still weary, I flipped over and dozed off again for however long it might last. You have no idea how absolutely wonderful it is to be able to simply lay down and sleep unless you have been deprived of it for months on end.

Without a doubt, my revival was hitting full stride.

As things progressed, rather than beginning each morning by automatically dumping another Boost down my tube, these days I was more inclined to fire up the stove and make a legitimate breakfast. It still hurt badly to swallow, but it seemed worth it. One morning I prepared a nice one-egg omelet with some bacon and cheese and along with that poured a large glass of V-8 juice (but you already knew that) and headed to the living room where I turned on the television and adjusted the volume so I could hear today's news. Finished with breakfast, I moved back to the kitchen and stood in the doorway for an extended gaze at the scattered medical supplies and prescriptions littering the place. If I expected to move onward toward full recovery this mess needed to change so I grabbed a sizeable plastic bag and tossed all the pills and liquids into it and set it aside for Karen to take into work and dispose of. Next I tidied up other areas of concern so our kitchen looked like a kitchen again. Lastly I retrieved a tiny aspirin and a vitamin E capsule and took them orally, just like in the olden days when there was no cancer or narcotics. So I guess if one seeks a definable moment this would be a good place to site a change in attitude that would lead to a more determined ascent up the other side and finally away from the pit of hell.

One by one the little victories added up. Eating became more and more doable, my voice eventually broke free, I discovered I could at last sleep on my sides, I slipped my headphones back over my ears and adjusted the volume up to where it belongs when twin fiddles play, and when I began pulling little pranks on Audrey and Karen anyone around here could see a renewed and rising hope seized the day—recovery was fully underway.

Lifelines

Patients saddled with the fight against cancer rapidly inherit two terminologies, Support and Team, both which will follow them wall-to-wall during their battle, and probably longer. Maybe it's just me, but I perceived two different lifelines; one I called personal support—well wishes, encouragement, and prayers from family, friends, or any number of possible acquaintances; and the other of course stemmed from professional support—the day in and day out assistance, monitoring, and tough love from doctors, nurses, and technicians.

It seems quite clear that a major goal toward helping those with cancer is to try to alleviate their tendency to feel alone. The instant you hear the word cancer you pull to the side of the road while the normal world continues to speed by. It is a very isolated feeling at first. But you are not alone. I hope most cancer stricken patients share a common experience to mine once I decided to publically divulge my plight. The initial outpouring of encouragement provided such positive energy it would come back to comfort me even during the darkest times. Even during the time when I chose to turn the world off for a while I made it a point to remember the magnitude of personal support waiting in my corner once I was able to break my seclusion.

Having now seen and felt cancer from up close I want to talk about a certain matter of personal support that would understandably be harder to grasp from otherwise caring well-wishers. Once treatments began to weaken me I turned more guarded and when a cancer patient takes that turn, personal support can prove to be a double-edged sword. On the downslide I began coughing badly and my throat felt, of course, like sandpaper much of the time. Salivary glands began shutting down and then, of course, it marked rock bottom when I realized I could no longer assume a lying down posture without igniting dry-heaves and coughing so abrasive and convulsive I feared I would do permanent damage beyond what the treatments were already inflicting. Finally, one morning I awoke to find my voice would not work... at all. Zero. You really cannot blame someone for not wanting to be seen in such a condition, and truthfully I did not want others to know how bad it had gotten.

During this time I had a few friends who sought to go above and beyond. One important thing I learned is that cancer patients sometimes want nothing to do with visitors, text-messages, or phone calls—anything demanding immediate or sustained responses. Frustrated and discouraged by the mass exodus of my once positive frame of mind, upbeat persona, and supposed toughness, I now wanted nothing to do with anyone.

To say cancer treatments aren't pretty pars calling the Titanic a "boating accident." A typical cancer patient's self-image is quickly devastated. Sleep deprivation, perpetual fatigue, rapid physical deterioration, mental exhaustion, and fear, all take a toll. Surely a person in such disarray is not inclined to entertain a supportive chat at this point; they know mirrors don't lie. Cancer is a super-depressant, and the deeper into treatments the patient goes, probably the better it is for friends to leave them alone. Trust spouses or close family members to carry the ball through this phase. If you want updates on the patient, contact the spouse or family members, but remember, too, they are also sharing some of the burdens. No need to show them how concerned you are every two days.

139

Generally, given today's social media, you can be included on a list of people receiving updates on the patient. Usually the frequency of postings will differ according to the sensitivity of whatever interval the patient is in. In most cases, expect along the way to find a long interim of silence. Don't interrupt it. Just know the patient will never forget you are thinking about them and are pulling for them—believe me, we do know it and appreciate it to no ends.

One well-meaning friend kept asking about making baked goods for me even as I explained I was feeding via a tube drilled into my stomach; and even worse I got wind of another hatching a plan for an onsite celebration at the Cancer Center on the final day of my treatments. She wanted to hire a clown or magician, something along that order. I have already spoken about how out of place such a display would be, at least in my eyes, but without having the same experiences I was having, it is understandable that these friends would seek to do something like that. After all, they are among the finest and most compassionate friends I have. The last thing I mean to do is belittle the merits of their innocent intentions, but speaking now as one who has seen cancer firsthand it is always best to temper personal support to fit the circumstances and sometimes that means do nothing at all. I promise you, the patient knows who is thinking of them and knows who is in their corner.

During my own battle, there came a time early on when I could still manage some yard work, but not enough. My home landscaping is very important to me so I asked my brother and an ex-employee if they would be good enough to come up for a few hours on a Saturday and help me get the place in decent shape. My brother, Ron, brought his wife, Cheryl, along, ex-employee Nate showed up, Karen pitched right in, and I did what I could to hobble here and there and help out. After four hours we called it good, Karen cooked a nice lunch for all the helpers, and one could not sight a better example of personal support.

Slowly, though, I continued to erode and one day thinking I could still get at some of the yard work myself I fired up my backpack leaf blower but after just a few minutes wound up vomiting so badly I became light headed and nearly bit the dust. I gathered myself, returned to the basement to put my blower away and from that point on the stark sobering fact that I no longer functioned as anything but a cancer patient hit home. Soon enough, as I began to slide further, the only support to whom I would allow clearance were Karen and my professional team. One morning I showed up for treatments and Mike, the radiation tech, came to the lobby to escort me back for my treatment. After we left the lobby Mike turned to me and said, "I think I'm going to have the doc take a look at you before we go in this morning."

I knew right away what that meant.

It had grown apparent to my team down at the Cancer Center that I needed a short break. I didn't want a break, as that just stretched the process yet further, but I had promised to trust them and, really, what other choice did I have?

To be completely fair, they turned out correct in their assessment. Two days later in the early hours of the morning is when I wound up in the Emergency Room mentioned earlier. The coughing and dry-heaves had become uncontrollable. Unable to speak, I typed into my iPhone some brief symptoms and begged someone to please get me stabilized.

They spent several hours trying to decide what might be happening, took lung x-rays, checked for influenza, infused me with fluids to get me hydrated, but finally a doctor came in, sat next to me, and placed a comforting hand over my wrist.

"I'm guessing it's the treatments taking quite a toll Mr. Page. You're at the apex of a worst case scenario. You've been through a lot but at least the end is in sight."

By then I felt better than when I had arrived early that morning so didn't argue when he said he would rather not admit me to the hospital. Remember, too, this is the same doc that by chance happened to prescribe codeine, and I am quite certain codeine had much to do with my ability to finally put temporary holds on the coughing, particularly late into the nights.

Karen drove me home where by now it had grown customary for me to crawl daily into an entirely reclusive state. I didn't want to hear voices, I didn't want to see daylight, I closed my eyes and let time pass. Each night I waited for Karen to come in the door and that would brighten what could be brightened. Later at night when she would head off to bed I would try to read a bit, a couple e-books I had downloaded a while back knowing there would probably be time that needed killing, but after a chapter or two I would close down, wrap up in my blanket and sit in the darkness... another day gone.

Good.

Rock bottom lingered long enough for sure, but never did I feel so despondent that I would have given up. With Karen there to drive me to treatments and with her back at home each night, that alone provided enough fuel to hang tough and to always, always, keep envisioning days ahead when the outlook would not be so bleak, and perhaps not bleak at all; days ahead when a lifetime would resume wherein a cancer patient emerges good as new. Never once did I fall into such desperate retreat that I would doubt those days ahead. I will always believe the main reason to keep the faith had everything to do with the lifeline of support I knew would be waiting once I could pick myself back up. But at my lowest point, I rejected any immediate contact, withdrew from social media, left emails and personal messages unattended, and guessed it best that there be no such thing as an outside world until I could regain my bearings. Karen would tell me later that even during our drives to daily treatments my demeanor could not be breeched. And when I tried to bluff friendliness to anyone I crossed at the Treatment Center I could tell they were onto me. It was plain as day the Roger they had met in the beginning had vacated, but still they reciprocated with warmth and smiles while the more intricately involved, docs, nurses, and techs, took extra time to tell me how far I had come and how close I was to the end. Everything they had promised at the outset fell into place exactly as they said it would and even during those challenging days, on my last legs with a little over a week to go to fulfil my treatment schedule, I fully trusted them to see that I made it across the finish line should it come down to that.

Those were the hardest of days but as I said earlier, never did I doubt brighter ones ahead. A few weeks after my treatments were over, I began to rise from the pit of hell and inch my way up the other side. The further up I made it the more I beckoned again to personal support and again my friends did not let me down. I returned to posting weekly updates to social media and a core of reliable friends would take time to read the posts that I admit got lengthy, and their comments helped pull me along. I could never thank all of those people enough, but none of them would ask it, anyway. The difference makers were in full force for me the instant I called back out—I knew they were always there, even when I wasn't. That is the essence of overwhelming support that will aid every cancer patient that ever needs to lock horns in the fight for their tomorrows.

Everyday Difference Makers

When NFL great Jim Kelly presented the concept of difference makers he intentionally emphasized that his message be aimed at the most ordinary of us. The more of us who stay cognizant of the phrase and keep our eyes peeled for situations where a difference maker is needed the more the philosophy driving the phrase will permeate. The philosophy is of the essence. Each individual act on its own weighs differently depending on the magnitude of a situation; but the philosophy is already of the highest magnitude.

The philosophy behind being a difference maker suggests that our acts might cumulate into infectious behavior. That's why Kelly is so emphatic on pointing out that we do not need to be an Aaron Rodgers or Russell Wilson to make a difference. It is also why he opens the parameters to reach far and wide beyond the realm of cancer. Being a difference maker might be as simple as mowing your neighbor's lawn while they are away on vacation or lending aid to a person transferring from a wheelchair into a passenger's seat at the curb. Of course it can also mean hanging off a cliff to rescue a desperate mountain climber or landing a jetliner successfully on the Hudson River saving all aboard. The difference making I'm talking about though, is the simpler everyday stuff. It starts there. It is hardly a new philosophy, I get that, but it is hardly an overly played one, either. Maybe if I show you some of the people I have crossed paths with over these past months it will emphasize my point. Keep in mind none of these people are Aaron Rodgers or Russell Wilson, no, the difference makers I am going to show you are everyday people who are among us at all turns.

Way back on the day of my biopsy, a customer of mine from years back, Dianne, who volunteers at the hospital, spied me at the receptionists desk and her eyes widened in surprise.

"Roger, what on earth are you doing here?"

When I revealed my plight she nodded knowingly and said softly, "Me too, breast cancer."

"How are you doing with it?" I asked.

"Oh, I guess I'm going to be okay. The docs say I'm clean, but the treatments sure weren't fun."

When she learned more specifically about my cancer she told me about a friend of hers who had contended nearly the identical situation. She warned of horrible days ahead but then she smiled and said, "He's been okay now for six years. Back to eating too well," she laughed. "I know you. You'll beat this," she smiled.

When I introduced her to Karen, she said lightheartedly, "You make sure he does what he's told." Then out of the blue she added, "You married a good one with this guy," and I was glad for Karen to hear that from someone besides me. Ha.

So Dianne, fresh off her own bout with breast cancer, is volunteering at a hospital and is as upbeat as always—an everyday difference maker.

When I sent letters or emails out to my lawn care customers to inform them of my upcoming challenges, one of them, Arlene, replied with a lengthy response chronicling her battle versus a cancer very similar to mine. Her response warned me to prepare for the fight of my life, but softened the gloom with enough encouragement to assure me that in the end I should emerge whole again. Having worked for her for several years I was stunned to know she had fought such a battle. One thing about Arlene is her nonstop enthusiasm toward physical outdoor work. I am guessing her to be into her seventies, yet she still mows her large lawn with a push mower, keeps the shrubs trimmed up nicely, the gardens tended, and after all that she takes off on an extended hike around the neighborhood; so tell me what more a new patient readying for the unknown could ask for as far as a promising example of the "other side." If Arlene had waded through the pit of hell and back and was now firing on all eight with such envious zeal, surely I could look forward to that myself. Arlene is an everyday difference maker.

Another customer, Mary Beth, has sure seen her share of cancer treatments but appears to be on the other side. I've never really asked. But her response in learning about my upcoming battle was stark, honest, blunt, and to the point. If ever one were to wear the crown of "nobody lied," it is Mary Beth. She is the only one on earth that never talked about beating this or kicking its ass or how strong I was, no, she spoke right in the voice of cancer and forced me to hear some needed advice, and even warnings. Emphatically she urged me to listen to the medical pros, comply with all medications, and to always remember the friendliest four-letter-word in my near future will be rest. Her letter spanned two full pages of preparation, all of it bore true.

As you would expect, most customers took time to send me well wishes and the general tone carried a certain sophistication parring Arlene's and Mary Beth's. I appreciated reading them all, but in a refreshing contrast, one customer named, Bonnie, sent a card that took its own route in centralizing the theme of straight talk. "I know your luck sucks," she wrote, "but you'll make it."

From that point on, anytime Karen and I needed to lighten the atmosphere with a good laugh, I simply repeated Bonnie's sentiments and the world felt straightened back out. So, yes, Bonnie, in her own improbable way, winds up an everyday difference maker.

Two particular days which I have previously shared with you helped immensely in molding my faith in everyday difference makers: The day when my brother, his wife, and my ex-employee Nate came up to help out on the landscaping; and the day when we wound up buried by a formidable dumping of early snow in November.

To see the landscaping crew chattering and laughing away while they sheared shrubbery, pulled weeds, raked leaves and even mowed and trimmed the grass was very uplifting. Sure, it was only for a few fleeting hours, but I will treasure the lasting images of that day forever.

And when that November snow came dumping down and I watched it pile up and I wondered how I might hold up against it, I could never have imagined the difference makers that would touch my life the minute I dared walk out there with my oversized shovel and my oversized confidence. The instant I plunged my shovel into the compacted frozen mess out by the road I knew my efforts would not bode well. But now, and for the rest of my life, the eternal image of neighbor Joyce hustling up the road toward me, will be mine to drift back upon whenever I need a smile. Having dropped her own work midstream, her act of kindness triggered her husband to follow suit bringing a backhoe up to address the otherwise insurmountable packed mass out by the road. The increased activity caught neighbor Dale's eye as he came down the road in his truck where he slowed to a crawl and hollered out that he would be back soon with his snow-blower. And if all that wasn't enough, when I turned to sit down on the tailgate of one of my trucks for a breather, there came Karen scooping her way out to us with her bargain-bin eager-beaver little shovel to lend a hand as well. Do you see how forceful one simple act can turn out to be? Joyce, Jim, and Dale have been exceptional neighbors and I would never have thought one way or another had they not pitched in to help out that day. But that they *did* pitch in to help makes all the difference. With a simple decision to be a difference maker, Joyce headed up the hill to help a sick neighbor out.

That one kind act ignited just a few hours of compassionate concern, but those hours will last me a lifetime.

Every last one of us is capable of spawning the same chain reaction and the more of us who become cognizant of it will likely set into motion better days for our world's current and ongoing cultural failings. From what I have witnessed and felt during the past months, it is clear that most human hearts beat with a purpose that exceeds the self. There is a certain gratification in changing the look in another's eye if only for a moment. To lift another's spirit, to see a smile break through, to hear a gracious, "Thank you," all of these acts evolve from a basic human kindness that indeed exists in most of us.

Tammy works a custodial job down at the Corning Cancer Center. I presume she boasts none of the refined skills of the receptionists, nurses, doctors, technicians, or office clerks, throughout the facility where she pushes her cleaning cart. But there is not one soul, however polished or practiced, that frequents the entire Corning Hospital property, and probably for miles beyond, who could light up a room with a smile like Tammy's. When I began showing up at the Cancer Center, I, too, could flash quite a convincing smile and Tammy and I got to know each other as, "Smiley." Even at my lowest point when I couldn't make a sound or muster much more than a meek wave, Tammy held the fort for both of us by calling out, "Hi Smiley," whenever we saw each other. If Tammy can be such a determined difference maker, so can all of us.

I could never begin to mention them all, but each day I found myself lifted a bit by difference makers wall-to-wall in that treatment facility. One of my chemotherapy nurses, Bobbi, bought my books to give to her husband for Christmas, Doris, another whose mere smile uplifts a room, Latrice who continuously worked to keep my schedule straight, no problem or snafu worth mentioning, she would have it solved in no time, and receptionists Mary and Kelly were always friendly, efficient, and accommodating. Another receptionist, Lisa, whom I spoke of earlier doling out the red cards, is the first person I struck up a conversation with down there back on day one and the last one I waved goodbye to on my way out the door following my final treatment. The next time she saw me was a month-and-a-half later when I came in for an appointment and ambushed her by saying right out loud, "Well hello Lisa. How's it going?"

"You can talk!" she sighed, happily. "Listen to you!"

Each person in that facility cares deeply about the patients. Every last one of them are difference makers.

I haven't stopped to wonder how drawn I would have become to the phrase had I not so suddenly wound up one in need. I have always considered myself conscientious and polite, and have always tried to help others when it seemed appropriate, but to what degree? Now, having felt the compassion from so many people, so many angles, it is engrained within me to forever stay alert for any situation where I can make a difference.

Be it a kind word or act, always go at it knowing how much it would mean to *you* if the roles were reversed... because there will be times in all our lives when that will indeed be the case. Don't wait to get cancer to find it out.

Finally a day came, January 18, where at eleven o'clock in the morning I would come back around to a meeting with good ol' Sam and what I hoped to be a conclusive PET CT scan. You remember Sam from way back on day one, a man surrounded every day of his life by the threat of cancer, his lymphoma in remission, yet each day he involves himself with helping others through their own battles. Seeing Sam and his assistant Doug again after seven months seemed to take this part of the course full circle. No matter what the scan revealed I had made it this far and felt abound with confidence, much of it due to the ceaseless efforts of everyday difference makers that worked on my behalf, many of them knowing not a single thing about me other than I needed their help.

On the day of the scan I returned to my friends on Facebook. Say what you will about social media but it is where I found my largest assembled group of difference makers whom I could count on whenever I reached out. Regardless of how the scan might turn out, my feelings toward so many who had stayed the course with me would never change. It was important to me to tell them how I felt.

As far as complete recovery I have a ways to go. But mostly about my recovery, I have certainly reaped more than my share of support by reaching out to you guys over the course of this long haul. For those who have reached back to provide for me a lifeline bridging the past several months to a day when I might be well again, you have been the difference makers to whom I am permanently indebted and I will never forget it. Thank you beyond measure for your words of encouragement, prayers, and your many generous acts of kindness. And although I rarely see merit in applying the grossly overused word, "awesome," your support has proven to be just that in helping me get to this day. In a lifetime left, I will never be able to thank you enough.

After posting my sentiments Karen chauffeured me down to the hospital and I underwent the scan. Afterward I looked in on Karena and Doc Collier to say hello and to thank them again now that I could do it out loud. I spent extra time exchanging pleasantries with Lisa, telling her I expect a birthday card next May, and then Karen and I headed out the doors and into the parking lot. My step had regained its bounce, the air seemed fresher than ever, and to top it all off, as if on que, I suddenly heard a voice cry out from a ways off, "Hey Smiley!" Tammy, of course, her face beaming like rays of sunlight as she briskly made her way down the main walkway along the parking lot.

Seeing her like that and particularly at that point in time, seemed to thrust a dagger at an earache that evolved to rip open my eyes to the awful pain that can suddenly interrupt an otherwise excellent life. But on the count of, "Hey Smiley!" and the forever glowing face of Tammy, it came front and center out in that cold parking lot how much better off I in fact might actually wind up due to that earache of mine.

Most importantly to me about everyday difference makers, there is Karen. Looking back to Rodney Crowell's lyrics on the opening page of this book, to say there were turns where I would spin is quite an understatement, hell, sometimes I couldn't see a turn coming. But spin I did. Upon each turn throughout the unknown I spun in circles of confusion, fright, and even desperation. But not once did the stabilizing weight of a loving hand on my shoulder waver—not once. From start to finish, without asking anything of her, I received everything from her. That's just the way she's wrapped. Even considering this earache that escalated into a trip through hell and back, I would feel foolish to bemoan my luck. What I have in her, luck is not vast enough to explain. She loves me as I do her and if my life should end tomorrow I would far prefer to have lived a shortened life with both her and cancer, than to have lived a long life with neither.

The "Other Side"

I know I described cancer as pulling to the side of the road, but that's probably the polite version of omitting the part about smashing into a guardrail while you're at it. Suddenly appointments littered my calendar and anything heretofore resembling a happy semi-retirees relaxed schedule bit the dust. Off to see so and so in this or that office and with a port installed, a tube protruding, and a mesh mask fitted to my face my body took on the look of a weird science project. All through the preparation the swelling of the lymph node increased along with the pain while I grew more and more impatient to get these treatments started so I could begin my quest for the "other side." The "other side" was a phrase I heard almost immediately upon meeting with medical pros—that and the pit of hell. They all used it, the nurses, docs, techs, even the receptionists referred to the other side in cases like mine. Unlike terminal cases, the one saving grace in my condition was this repeated promise of the other side.

Had I given fitting credence to what it would take to get there I might not have been so eager to begin, but that, of course, is foolish. The longer you wait to get started the longer you take to get there and the trip is no less agonizing.

I have tried my best so far to give you a genuine map of the landscape but frankly have worn my own self out talking about the bottom. What I want cancer patients who are granted a chance at the other side to know is that one way or another you will climb free.

The tears will dry, the violent symptoms of a compromised body will dissipate, the anger will subside, depression won't last, and however low you feel, there is always, always, a turning point lying not far up ahead. Cry, swear, sulk, and cry some more, but keep knowing there is a turning point coming.

To be honest, even recognizing my own turning point and seizing it was not much of an ultimate victory. But I did indicate the return of a cognizant thought process and the game I invented simply asked, "was this day a little better than yesterday?" Most days the answer was yes and some days that "yes" rang more convincingly than others; but most days got a little bit better in one way or another—welcome to The Other Side.

I haven't climbed high enough up the other side yet to get a gauge on how long it takes to make it to the upper flats where a patient can stand completely upright, peek back over the ridge and sigh, "I cannot believe I made it up outta there." My guess, if you really want to know, is never. The scars of having cancer probably do not ever entirely heal. Even should a patient reach a point where they are labeled, "clean," there is the residual anxiety that I simply cannot believe ever goes away. When Sam first told me, "Cancer changes your life forever," I saw the chilling look in his eyes and felt it, too, in my own. I believe it word for word and believe I always will.

So when you put faith in this other side let's keep reality in play as well. Face it, "the other side" is an incentive based phrase and I think a darned good one. But here on the other side is not nearly the same as the place you came from before cancer. That place is forever gone, and wherever or how far your travels take you beyond the other side, cancer will forever dog your shadow.

But that is the wrong way to look at things and I know it is. From what I have seen of cancer patients, and those in the professional field combatting cancer, all seem up to the task of fortifying a fiery eyed defiance that serves to keep the peace. These days when I chew and swallow a savory piece of ribeye steak, or work my way through a magnificent slice of Aniello's pizza, or sip a heavenly caramel latte, I do so in comparison to days not long ago when life was sustained by a product called, Boost-Plus that I poured down a tube into my stomach. My throat was in such a way I could barely swallow water, and eventually I chose to even pour my liquids through the tube. But really, before cancer, the way I used to devour a ribeye steak or wolf a slice of pizza has no resemblance to how I do it now and I am pretty sure I will never again be able to eat that way. I am a culinary freak—love to cook special cuts of venison, concoct sauces that knock your hat in the creek, and I challenge anyone in the world to outdo me frying perch or bullhead fillets... anyone. I used to fry sixteen perch fillets at a time and eat them in two settings... sometimes one if I was showing off, ha. Most recently, though, I fried and ate four and then had four the following day. They were good to eat again, I hadn't tasted perch splattered with malt vinegar and sprinkled with salt in a long while. But in all honesty, they are nothing like in the olden days when the taste seemed more like an addiction. I miss those days, sure, but not nearly as much as I cherish these ones. That describes this "other side," as best I can. Any cancer patient yearns to get here, but to compare it from where you began... no.

The only fair way to view this "other side," is to compare it to where you could have wound up. Be thankful that in many cases cancer is not the death sentence it once was. Medicinally, this world has evolved in leaps and bounds. Research and Development continues to exceed expectations and more and more patients are reaching the other side.

Just to feel the chance again to hike with Audrey, to hunt deer, to rejoin the perch chase, to pitch magazine articles, to write and sell these books, to resume my livelihood in semi-retirement, to sit on the deck sipping hot, strong black coffee in the dark waiting for the first chirp from the first bird and watching for sunup, to spend hours upon hours tending my landscape here at home, to lounge about with Karen watching hockey or football games on television, to zoom off on ten-day vacations, is restoration enough. To feel again the worth of each breath we are granted is immeasurable.

And isn't there a pretty good chance for life to be even better once the threat of having it taken is resolved? I have never considered myself to be one who takes life for granted. I have always tried to reap the most from a day and have always kept my frame of mind aimed in positive directions. If that was the case before being subjected to a bout with cancer and being dragged and beaten through the pit of hell, how much might one's hopes be amplified when they finally pull themselves far enough up the other side to where their life resumes to be at least a fair semblance of how it once was? I can tell you without having yet felt it, that first tick of a biting perch is likely to stir quite a celebratory eruption. Just firing up that boat motor again is going to be a high and mighty middle finger to the pit of hell. So, yeah, I'll take life here on the other side for whatever it turns out to be and for however long it lasts. Each new sunrise begins a day that might not have come about without the encouragement derived from an endless chorus of voices promising the other side. Even as I crawled toward it blindly at times, just to know it existed substantiated that whatever efforts were required to make it would end up worth it. I now know each word of that rings true.

Resurgence

It felt good to feel good again, and especially to feel good about my chances for a full recovery. Although my appetite hasn't returned in full and eating is still a struggle at times, it at least drew clear enough for that the feeding tube should no longer be needed. I couldn't wait to hear that news from a doctor though at which point it would become official. If it was up to me the thing would have been gone long ago.

In fact, now, the only issue holding me back was due to throat issues, some lingering coughing fits and the annoyance of having to regurgitate at times in order to get food to go all the way down. I did worry that I wasn't consuming enough vegetables and essentially zero fruits but soon enough I should be able to get back on track with those. Many foods were back on the table, though, and I hoped for the best about increasing my appetite and intake. To be honest, my weight had plummeted too far. When this all began I was pushing three hundred pounds and disgusted about it so before any real activity toward fighting the cancer I had embarked on a rigorous campaign to drop some weight and in a very healthy way dropped nearly thirty pounds. The official starting weight used by Karena and Doctor Collier was two-sixty-eight. The demand was that I not lose ten percent of that weight or treatments would stop until I beefed back up. In my mind there was no way on earth I would lose twenty-seven pounds in two months, it seemed almost impossible. At my final weigh-in two days prior to my final treatment the scale read two-forty-two, almost exactly to the pound of a ten-percent drop. When I tell you I would probably not have made it another week I am not joking. My sleep deprived body limped on auto-pilot, no desire to eat, and my mental state had deteriorated so that I hardly recognized myself. But Karena and Doctor Collier each seemed confident I had at least two good days left in the tank, so they brushed the weight off and none of us mentioned it again.

The strange thing is, even as I continue to recover and feel better each day, my weight is reluctant to join the process. At its worst I had dropped all the way down to two-twenty-six, but as I write this in late January I have taken it back up to over two-thirty. But at two-hundred and thirty pounds these days, I sure as sin feel a whole lot stronger than I did at a weakened two-forty-two back in October. The truth is I aim to eventually weigh about two-thirty, that was the goal way back when I embarrassedly neared three-hundred pounds. But the two-thirty I want to weigh includes muscle tone in my arms and legs which will take some time to recoup.

So, yes, there is still some uphill left to cover, particularly in reconstructing a balanced diet. The problem is everything tastes salty. Whatever dominant forces are in play when it comes to taste have determined I must like salt. But I do not prefer salt on fruits, cereals, milk, ice-cream, green salads, and I could go on and on. I do eat an occasional green salad out of spite, but for the most part any food that I don't like salt on is not part of the curriculum yet. Now foods that I *do* like salt on, meats, sauces, pasta, casseroles, fish, poultry, potatoes, and things like that, the door is open. But always figured into the equation is a compromised throat and who knows how long it will take for that to ever return to something like normal. It still hurts to swallow, sometimes it hurts like hell, so I'm assuming that is playing at least a psychological role in my lack of appetite.

As far as my physical progress, there recently came another dumping of snow here in January, not quite as heavy as the one

166

back in November, but no walk in the park, either. I fetched my giant shovel and trenched my way out to the road to begin shoveling that heavy crap the road crews with their giant plows leave in their wake. Joyce and Jim left for Florida shortly after Christmas so that card wasn't in play and although I cannot say I felt worthy of Superman's cape by any means, I did slowly but surely dig my way through the mess. Once I got to the easier stuff, if that's ever a way to describe ten to twelve inches of snow, I was able to hang tough enough to shovel the driveway clear down to the vehicles. Neighbor Mike came over to pitch in and he helped me along during the final stretch and I was glad of it. But if snow is any indication I am gaining in leaps and bounds.

Remember, it wasn't long ago when I lacked confidence in seeing my sixty-fourth birthday. I'm new to cancer and all I heard at first is, "You are going to die." When more experienced people entered my life they were extremely honest and I have learned that cancer does demand honesty. Everyone I have met who is unwilling to simply pray it away has impressed me as exceptionally candid. When I decided to title the book, *Nobody Lied*, I hope to have captured what I have learned myself through the people I have met and what I can only describe as a brotherhood of bravery. I have also learned the great comradery that exists among cancer patients. Recently at a trade show I apologized to a broker about my voice, explained things and he said, "Yeah, me, too," and he described his own bout with cancer some fifteen years ago. These days the guy looks like a fitness instructor, not a boat salesman, but before parting he shook my hand and each of us patted the other on the shoulder and wished the other good luck. We'll never see each other again, but we will continuously come across our kind and each time follow the unwritten rule about the pats on the shoulder, the gentle hugs, and the misty eyes, because each knows what kind of bravery the other needed to employ just to be here today. To have weathered storms none of us would ever choose to combat must on a somewhat smaller magnitude par soldiers surviving wars. Once a person experiencing such fright and fear makes it through they emerge with a greater understanding and appreciation for life.

So far this chapter might not sound much like a patient's resurgence, but if you keep your eye on the ball you have to ask if I am not a better person due to cancer. Even as I wrote that it seemed insane, but in many ways the rest of my days, to know they might not have happened, should be even brighter and yet more fulfilling than those before cancer. I would stop short of calling myself lucky, but in making a positive from a negative it at least poses a sensible argument.

A couple things happened that will make you chuckle, maybe laugh outright, and I'm all for that.

First, regarding my resurgence, the instant I bit into that venison hotdog it rekindled hopes I would resume meat eating down the road. Those were still tender days, though, and it wasn't until a couple weeks later that I pressed more deeply by thawing out a package of one-inch-thick venison steaks. There were only three in the package and I fried just one at a time but in two days, all the steaks gone, I could fully assume that venison is back on the table.

The one glaring problem is I had forfeited the deer season. Once I realized I would just as soon add a deer to the freezer I put the word out to neighbor Mike, his cousin Pete and Pete's wife, Darlene. Should any of them find an extra deer lingering around their stands I could supply a tag for it and happily process it. By now, however, the best part of the season was over, we were late into gun season and the extra deer I hoped might venture forth never materialized. No biggie, I suppose, but with only a couple days left of muzzleloader season, which would conclude the 2018 deer hunt, a friend of mine sent a message on Facebook.

"Roger. Jeremy (her son) was asking if you would be able to use a deer if he could get one for you."

"YES."

"Okay. I'll let him know."

"Wow. Thank you."

"You bet."

And what do you know, on the final evening of the season I received a text message from Jeremy.

"Are your knives sharpened?"

Holy smokes, he'd come through on a nice plump doe.

Jeremy brought the doe to my basement where I love to process my own venison. He helped me hang the deer for skinning and processing and over the next two days amid happily butchering and packaging various cuts of meat I felt a sense of normalcy seeping back in.

Soon after finishing my deer, my determining PET CT scan loomed on the horizon but the way I was feeling indicated that no matter what the scan reveals I had better get in gear and ready up for some serious fishing. My boat motor had unfortunately sat idle for too long with gas remaining in the carburetor so there was that to tend to. I lugged it to motor mechanic Ross and pre-paid him, then zoomed right straight down to our local Field & Stream store nearby. In there I needed a couple new rods and a bunch of plastic jig bodies to get started on my new endeavor of fishing Keuka's lake trout from the depths. It is a fascinating way to fish. Using electronics you can watch the image of your heavy jig drop toward bottom where you can watch the images of interested fish begin to assemble or charge. I can't wait to get started. On the way home I stopped and gassed the truck up—hadn't had it out in a while, and the instant I got home I fired up my laptop and sat down to continue shopping. I found my jig heads by following directions of another fisher I had met last year. The heads would be made in a garage it looked like and paying for them required updating my account with PayPal. With that done I headed to the mecca FishUSA and rang up a few hundred dollars in new reels, braided lines, ice-fishing line, more plastics, and at checkout tossed in a couple of those cool FishUSA tee-shirts, too.

Okay, to be truthful, this Visa card had been lying pretty much at bay for the past couple months, I agree with that, but when I went to check out from FishUSA I received the oddest notice that the card's supplier refused the order.

What?

I tried again to the same result. This has never happened to me before; I'm as honest as the day is long when it comes to online shopping. What gives?

Plan B came clear enough. Rather than cancelling the intensive order and trying to reconstruct it later—I still had more shopping to do elsewhere—I quickly relied back to PayPal and selected the option of direct pay from Karen's and my bank account. There. Worked. Good.

The next stop was at a site another fishing friend had told me about and all I needed to pick up there was a four-hundred dollar portable sonar graphing system, the Humminbird Helix 5. At checkout my Visa custodians continued to monitor what they thought to be strange and suspicious activity so again told me no dice. Couldn't they tell this was *not* a random spree of a loose cannon pulling off an identity theft? It was all *fishing gear* for crime's sake—*entirely* understandable. Anyway, PayPal saved me again so I headed off to Ebay for the final purchases of a long shopping day, a cool line spooling tool and a spare eighteen pound anchor for my boat. Seeing the writing on the wall I went directly to PayPal to cover Ebay.

That evening Karen received an email, an inquiry from our bank's credit department asking her about the legitimacy of today's purchases. She took time to reply that, "Jeez, none of you guys must be married to a fisherman, for crying out loud..." but before she could get too elaborate I told her to let me call the next day to make sure I have it all straightened out.

Our banking staff is always congenial, they hire a bunch of lighthearted and fun people so I held nothing back when a Stephanie answered the phone with a pleasant tone, "Thank you for calling First Heritage, my name is Stephanie, how can I help you today?"

"You guys down there don't understand fishing for beans, do ya?" I spurted, intentionally.

Silence.

"I'm just kidding," I laughed, after leaving her stranded for a prolonged second or two. I then took time to explain my recovery process and admitted I had perhaps gotten a bit exuberant in my sudden shopping spree. By now Stephanie was laughing along as I continued to paint the picture of the resurrected fisher with a green light on goods, and I ended by promising to be more careful in the future.

For our own purposes, a deer hanging in the basement one day and a rambunctious credit card reeling in a bunch of fishing gear the next represents at least the strong confidence one might need to continue scaling the other side.

The Telling PET CT Scan

Friday January 18th finally arrived. One of Sam's assistants led me back to the scanner where Sam seemed cheerfully unsurprised by the way I greeted him, "Hi Sam. Don't screw this up."

Truthfully I would love to have an extended conversation with Sam someday, but it's impossible in the medical setting. I have learned enough about him though to know we would be good friends if it ever came to that. We are of the same age, a similar past, both cancer patients, and most of all we see things a lot alike.

The scan itself is always unremarkable. Afterward I took some time to wander about the Cancer Center to thank the people so instrumental in helping me through all of this. I hadn't been in the Cancer Center in quite some time; the protocol being to wait three months after the last treatment before undergoing the scan. Strange as it seems, it was good to visit the Center again; to see those faces again.

The following Thursday, January 24th, we met with Doctor Gosain to go over the results. I had confidently anticipated a clean slate, but in reality I don't think that ever again exists. There will always be worries and doubts for me as I press on to live the rest of my life the very best I can. In this case, although Doc Gosain smiled when he told me all three of the docs, himself, Doctor Collier, and Doctor Sussman, were unanimously "very pleased," with what they saw, he did indicate some remaining "activity" on the lymph node. The HPV carcinoma at the tongue base was gone, and the lymph node had dropped from an SUV value of 16.8 to 2.2 which I interpret as indicative it had taken a full hit, too. The "activity" explained Doc Gosain, could very well be scar tissue.

Of course, to my ears, anything but "all clear and clean," leaves me on pins and needles. Detecting my worry, Doc Gosain honed in like he can, squaring his eyes directly with mine and said, "What I want to know mostly is how do you feel."

"I feel like a million bucks," I replied honestly, "but I'll feel a lot better when there's no activity in that lymph node."

He understood and told me they would run a CT scan on February 15th and suspected my hopes would be granted.

175

Seeing the writing on the wall, that they're going to want to leave this tube in me, I added quickly to my response.

"The only other thing wearing its welcome out is this darned feeding tube, doc. I want it gone; is there any chance of that happening anytime soon?"

The plan, said Doctor Gosain, was to leave it in place for another six weeks "just in case," but my reaction to that was, "Doc, I haven't even needed to use it for the *past* six weeks." Then before I could stop myself, I blurted, "This thing is bullshit." The sincerity in which I spoke prompted Doctor Gosain to scrunch his face in a form of contending thought before he nodded, smiled, and said, "Let me talk with Doctor Collier and see what we can do. You've obviously seen enough of the tube."

"Yes. A long time ago."

"Okay, I'll get back with you today or early tomorrow."

"Thanks doc. I know how important this tube was, really I do. It saved my life. But I've just come to hate the thing. It limits everything I want to do."

"Okay, my friend, let me talk with Doctor Collier to be sure we're all on the same page."

That evening I received the news I could have the tube removed during my upcoming appointment with Jenn Cornish on February 7th. Longer than I want, but to have a hard date on its removal is otherwise music to my ears.

(*Also, that the docs would allow its removal just a week prior to a CT scan makes me believe they actually do believe the "activity" in the lymph node might not mean—Part Two.*)

Never The End

I want to end this here.

I've beaten us up enough and the next book I'm working on is about cruises so you really can't fault my desire to jump ship, ha.

What I have learned over these past months has increased my awareness ten-fold of what a magically wonderful life many of us are granted and how tragically some lives are cut short. If you are living a fulfilling life be thankful for each healthy breath but by all means stay aware, too, that it takes just the slightest earache to alter your course. While you are healthy, your calendar unblemished by weekly doctor appointments, your sleep augmented with sweet dreams, your appetite rounded and full, don't waste that. Get off your couches, turn off the television set, monitor the iPhone usage, and go places where you can breathe. Go places that make your eyes burst, go where your pulse races, go places where your palate erupts, or go places where in silence you can rest a minute to think about what a gift it is to live and breathe.

If your life is to be cut short, make sure you leave here knowing still what a great gift you were bestowed and that you made the most of it. There are people we all know who could live a thousand years and never see much of a day's worth. Don't be one of those. We all know, too, people who will not see another year, yet they lived to be a thousand. Be like them. Always be like them.

Once I began feeling better I wrote an article for Deer & Deer Hunting Magazine. Never have nine-hundred words so tidily spilled forth without much of a dot or dash needed in editing. I titled it, *Lessons Gained From A Season Lost*, and In accepting the article, editor Gordy Krahn replied, "*Nice piece, Roger. I'm looking forward to sharing it with DDH readers. Since you and I are the same age, this really hit home. Thanks for sharing. I am so glad to hear the good news that you are recovering well. Praying for a full recovery.*"

Having talked several times herein about difference makers it was at a very low point when Gordy, along with chief editor of Deer & Deer Hunting, Dan Schmidt, two extremely busy people, took time to dig up an old "Reader's Recoil" letter. Dan forwarded to Gordy who forwarded to me, "*Hey Roger, how are the treatments going? Thought you might enjoy this letter from one of our readers."*

He attached the following letter.

I was just reading Roger Page's recent article, "Ornaments," in Deer & Deer Hunting, and I have to admit that I cried. Here I am, a 60-year-old man crying. Roger could not have described the taking of an animal any better.

I have about 10 sets of antlers on my wall, and each of them have a story. I do not "decorate" my antlers and never will. These antlers and the stories behind the deer that were carrying them are too precious to me to have them covered up with decorations.

I wish this article would be published in every magazine. Come to think of it, copies of this D&DH article should be handed out with every hunting license so that every hunter would have to read it.

Timothy (last name withheld)
Owatonna, MN

Ornaments expressed my discontent whenever I see mounted animals decorated for the holidays. The diligent work of taxidermists sustaining a moment in time only to have their work covered with Christmas lights and Santa hats is appalling. It blatantly disrespects the animal, number one, it crudely decimates the refined skills of taxidermists, number two, but most of all it speaks to the hunter's own scruples and the self-respect they lack in allowing such frivolity.

Naturally I targeted the article for a December issue and it is plain to see that at least for one old hunter I wound up a prominent difference maker. I hope the article, in fact, touched a lot more readers in that way.

So even during some bleak days, Gordy, Dan, and Timothy from Minnesota, lifted my spirits and kept me believing in a day ahead when I could rejoin their ranks. I birddogged letter-writer Timothy's whereabouts and mailed him a signed copy of my book, "*A Hunter's Trail.*" He promptly and cordially responded as you would expect, proving that even in a world where cancer infiltrates, there are often beaten paths around it.

If this "activity" in the original lymph node winds up as the doctors think it will, I am ready for days in the woods, open waters, and full course meals; if not, I am ready for whatever they say is next. What I would not want to do is take a reader backward in any way at all. You have stayed with me through these pages despite my saying off the bat that it was with hesitance I dared even begin. I knew how roughly the pages were going to turn through chapters of darkness, sadness, and maybe even risking a desperate hopelessness at times as well. I hated every one of those pages.

But I knew, too, you were going to meet some of the most influential people on earth. I wanted you to know them as I do and I hoped all along that I might lead you through the necessary gloom to see the brightening horizon that is called the other side.

We are here and I feel it to be a good parting place.

Should the "activity" imply that I will be entering a phase two, I will see where it unfolds and keep silent about it until it seems wiser to speak. Right now, what I wanted you to see was a man snatched from a fulfilling life, thrown to the pit of hell, and I wanted you there each step of the way including the other side to prove we perhaps don't know our own capacity to survive. I wanted you to understand that, heaven forbid, if this ever happens to you, you will never need fear going it alone. I wanted you to understand that if cancer never affects your own life, you have no reason for leaving a single stone unturned once your time here is up. Cancer or not we are all terminal, one way or another, so the most important thing is to remember that the people who could have been here in your place, but will in fact never see the light of a single day, outnumber the grains of sand in the Arabian Desert.

I wanted you to challenge your perspective to make sure you are giving life a fair appraisal. I wanted to be sure that you oust boredom as if it's the devil; that you never wake up slowly but instead tear ass into each day before it happens that you wake up one morning to a subtle earache.

I wanted you to meet difference makers and more than that wanted you to see it in yourself. It's there.

I wanted you to meet the medical pros and to show you what outstanding human beings are there for us when we pull to the side of the road. I wanted you to bear witness firsthand of what we are all capable of no matter how low we plummet. I wanted you to see the pit of hell without feeling its wrath but to know if you are ever mandated to take it on, you will win. You *will win.*

I never wanted to have cancer. I never want you to have cancer. But I want more than anything else in the world to have taken you on a trip that shows you what an incredible gift we have in life, and among whatever hurdles mar our way I want you to know you are stronger than you can ever imagine.

For me, who knows? The "activity" might be put to rest and gone by mid-February; or it might open a floodgate toward an entirely new fight. Either way, count on me to thrive as best I can and to never forget what I have gained, even amid the lousy lows and especially amid the rejuvenating recovery.

As far as a happy ending goes? I honestly believe all the authors in the world combined throughout history could write thousands upon thousands of pages and never find a way to a happy ending about cancer. Already I have learned there will never be a full recovery—ever. There has never lived a cancer patient who rides happily into a glowing sunset glimmering beneath a romantic arching rainbow promising the world's brightest tomorrow. There is never the end. Cancer patients live day by day wondering when the next "activity" brings up questions that might send them back to treatments and even if it never happens that way it lingers as fear of the dark must. But what I have learned since being a cancer patient is to live each new day fully. That's all.

Here at the end of our road together, I ultimately see my own travels aimed forth into the unknown... or I should say, further yet into the unknown. But one thing is clear enough. I will travel more as a brother of humanity than I once did. I will stop and make a difference when called upon. I will spit in cancer's eye as best and often as I can, and if I emerge a better person from it day by day I will consider it to be a happy enough ending.

As we part and say goodbye here I will linger for a awhile if it's alright, and look after you as you disappear down your own road. It would mean so much to know that you go forth a better person from reading this short book. I want to picture you leaving here as a difference maker. I want our brief time spent together to have mattered.

More than anything else, I want to always be remembered as your friend.

So long.

The Author

Roger Page, sixty-three years old, is eager to get past cancer and back to enjoying semi-retirement after thirty-one years of operating a landscaping business. Part of his semi-retirement found him embarking on a second career in outdoor writing. You can find his articles frequently on the pages of *Deer & Deer Hunting Magazine*. Over the past few years he has also landed articles in *North American Whitetail, Bear Hunting Magazine, Life In The Finger Lakes, New York Game & Fish,* and *Fur-Fish-Game.*

He wrote his first two full-length books—*An Improbable Cast... Called Fishing Partners*, and *A Hunter's Trail—Steps Well Chosen*, in keeping with his favorite genres. Since then he has answered calls of duty with a book about landscaping—*The Landscape Tamed*, and now, of course, the book you have just finished that came about unexpectedly. His fifth book, a happier one indeed, all about Caribbean cruises should complete enough of an arsenal to hit the road with. Hopefully there is such a thing as a book show circuit where the objective will be less about selling books and more about meeting and blabbing with people like you.

All of Page's books can be found and purchased from Amazon.

With any luck cancer will not further infringe upon the author's love for the outdoors where he hunts passionately, fishes more passionately, and loves his goofy hounds to no ends. Most of all he loves his wife of thirty-seven years, Karen, and their rural life in Addison, NY.

www.ingramcontent.com/pod-product-compliance
Lightning Source LLC
Chambersburg PA
CBHW051310220526
45468CB00004B/1290